Spirometry

José Almirall, MD, MSc, PhD

Copyright © 2017 José Almirall

All rights reserved.

ISBN-13: 978-1546312963
ISBN-10: 154631296X

DEDICATION

I consider this book the product of a learning process for many years that started when I was a medical student. Upon its writing, repeatedly came to my mind the names of those who, in one way or another, participated in my training and shaped my understanding of the respiratory system: Milic, Ñico, Alex, Peter, David. All of them physicians, teachers, and researchers in the respiratory field. Without their combined influence this book would have not been possible. It is dedicated to them.

PREFACE

It is well known that lung functionality cannot be adequately evaluated relying only on symptoms referred by patients or a clinical exam. This occurs because mild pulmonary disease may be present with few symptoms, and may develop without the existence of signs indicating its presence. The use of spirometry may be of great help in this situation.

Spirometry may help in the early detection of respiratory problems in asymptomatic patients or may improve the care of patients known to have respiratory diseases. In principle, spirometry is a simple technique. However, concerns about properly using the technique and adequately interpreting test results are frequent among health professionals.

This book is intended to help in the use of spirometry. The book is divided in two parts. The first part deals with general aspects of the spirometry technique, and contains information and descriptions intending to provide the reader a general idea of the technique. The second part is dedicated to test interpretation, and is intended to be a guide in the process of understanding the significance of the numeric results.

Hopefully, the book may help to overcome barriers preventing a more widespread use of spirometry.

J.A

CONTENTS

PART 1 General aspects of the technique   1

Chapter 1 Spirometry and spirometers   3

  Spirometry   3

  Spirometers   5

Chapter 2 What do we measure with spirometry?   11

  Pulmonary ventilation   11

  Limitations of spirometry   14

  Spirometry tests   15

    Static lung volumes   15

    Minute ventilation   18

    Maximal voluntary ventilation   20

    Forced expiration   22

    Forced inspiration   25

Chapter 3 Forced expiration: parameters and performance   29

  Parameters measured from the forced expiratory volume-time curve   29

    Forced vital capacity (FVC)   29

    Forced expiratory volume in time interval t (FEVt)   31

Forced expiratory flow between 25% and 75% of the forced vital capacity (FEF25-75%)	32
Forced expiratory volume (timed) to forced vital capacity ratio (FEVt/FVC)	34
Parameters measured from the forced expiratory flow-volume curve	35
Peak expiratory flow (PEF or PEFR)	35
Forced expiratory flow related to some portion of the FVC curve (FEFx)	36
Performance of the test of forced expiration	37
Exclusion spirometry	39
Test of forced expiration without spirometer	40
Chapter 4 Variability in spirometry	**43**
Biologic variation	44
Intra-individual variability	44
Inter-individual variability	44
Variation due to dysfunction or disease	45
Variation due to airway obstruction	45
Variation due to restriction of lung excursion	46
Variation due to a mixed abnormality	46

PART 2 Spirometry interpretation   49

Chapter 5 General aspects of spirometry interpretation   51

    Graphic results   52

    Numeric results   56

Chapter 6 What do all these numbers mean?   59

    Reference (predicted) values   59

    Lower limits of normal   60

    Spirometry patterns   61

    Spirometry patterns with reduced FVC   62

    Obstructive spirometry patterns   66

    Isolated FEV_1 reduction   70

    Severity classification of ventilatory impairments in spirometry   72

Chapter 7 Bronchodilator response   75

    Persistent airway obstruction after a bronchodilator test   79

Chapter 8 Interrelationship of spirometry parameters: a graphical approach   81

Chapter 9 Interrelationship of spirometry parameters: global lung function 2012 reference values   93

Chapter 10 Interrelationship of spirometry parameters: practical implications   87

Chapter 11 Step by step analysis of numeric results   109

Chapter 12 Interpretation exercises   119

    Exercise 1   120

    Exercise 2   121

    Exercise 3   122

    Exercise 4   123

    Exercise 5   124

    Exercise 6   125

    Exercise 7   126

    Exercise 8   127

    Exercise 9   128

    Exercise 10   129

References   131

Appendix. BTPS correction   137

Index   139

PART 1

GENERAL ASPECTS OF THE TECHNIQUE

José Almirall

Chapter 1

SPIROMETRY AND SPIROMETERS

The prefix **spiro** comes from the Latin word *spirare*, which means to breath. Considering the root of the word, a definition for spirometry is the act or process of measuring breathing. A spirometer or spirograph is the instrument used for measuring breathing.

Spirometry

The language is constantly in evolution and the meaning of some words changes with time. When Jonathan Hutchinson started the modern phase of spirometers,[1] spirometry meant only the measurement of what is known today as vital capacity (the maximum volume of air exhaled from the point of maximum inspiration), and a spirometer was an inverted sealed cylinder floating on water which measured only volume. Since then, the meaning of spirometry has changed and spirometers have greatly been improved. An important improvement to spirometers was the recording of volume changes with time. One way to do this was using mechanical devices such as a pen attached to a system that followed the upward and downward movements of a cylinder floating on water (Figure 1-1). The pen could draw the cylinder's movements on a drum rotating at a constant speed (kymograph). This way, the spirogram (in this case the volume-time spirogram) or recording of breathing was obtained with a spirometer. This innovation allowed making other spirometry tests and the measurement of new parameters. At that point, spirometry meant much more than just measuring vital capacity. With continuous technical advances, electronic devices were added to spirometers and this led to the introduction of the measurement of instantaneous flow. This led to the measurement of even more spirometry parameters.

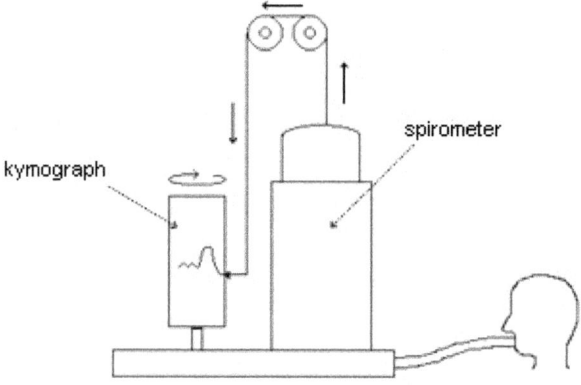

Figure 1-1. Schematic representation of a sealed-cylinder type spirometer with a rotating drum (kymograph) where a pen records the upward and downward movements of the cylinder.

The possibility of measuring instantaneous flow not only expanded the number of new parameters that could be measured to quantify the spirogram, but also allowed introducing another way of recording the spirogram: the flow-volume curve. All these innovations quickly moved from research to clinical laboratories and practice. With time, spirometry utilization in medical practice produced a sort of 'natural selection' of tests and parameters more often used. Reproducibility and simplicity were important factors determining the selection. This way, the test of forced expiration, i.e. a test in which the subject inspires to his/her maximal lung volume, then blows out as forcefully as possible and keeps expiring to as low a lung volume as possible, has been preferred over other tests. The extensive use of the test of forced expiration has made this test the symbol of spirometry. In our days, many studies applying spirometry only use this test. The simplicity and reproducibility of the test of forced expiration along with the availability of good portable spirometers have allowed applying the test at different levels of health care, from pulmonary function laboratories in hospitals to the bedside of patients. For its usefulness and frequent clinical application, this work is focused on the test of forced expiration. When mentioning spirometry, this book refers to the test of forced expiration, except in chapter 2 where other spirometry tests are briefly described.

Spirometers

Spirometers may be classified according to the primary measurement they make. Classically, two main groups are considered: volume-sensing devices, and flow-sensing devices. In our days, the majority of spirometers are of the flow measuring type due to their small size and relatively low cost.

The volume-sensing devices are based on primary measurements of the volume of air from which flow data are derived. In these devices, air is inhaled from and exhaled in a calibrated container to measure volume (Figure 1-1). Then, the flow rate can be calculated by electronic processing of the volume data (Figure 1-2).

The calibrated container used to measure volume could be either an inverted sealed cylinder or a wedge-shaped container floating on water, or a moveable piston or bellows. The minimal standards that these devices should meet in order to make reliable measurements have been described in detail elsewhere and the interested reader is referred to that publication for information regarding this matter.[2]

The volume displacement spirometer should be calibrated and meet the performance standards for the tests for which it is to be used. A common source of error in volume-sensing spirometers can be an air leak at any point in the tubing or apparatus.

Leakage may occur at the mouthpiece, a perforated or cracked bell or bellows, or through an insufficient level of water in a water spirometer. Leaks can be detected when performing consecutive maneuvers and a consistent displacement of the curves is observed.

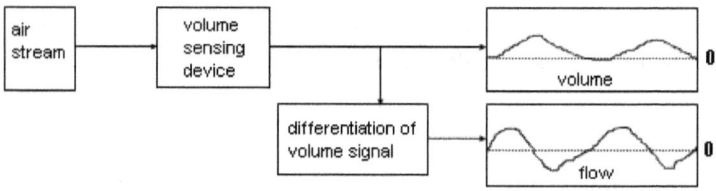

Figure 1-2. Diagram showing the steps followed to obtain volume and flow signals with a volume-sensing device.

Flow-sensing devices are called pneumotachographs, pneumotachometers or anemometers. They are placed directly in the air stream to sense airflow, and the volume data is obtained by electronic processing of the flow signal (Figure 1-3). Several types of pneumotachographs have been developed based on different physical principles. These principles include, among others, differential pressure flow through a resistance, rate of cooling of a heated wire, and rate of rotation of a turbine. The application of each principle has its own technical problems which are addressed by the makers of the devices to reflect accurately the instantaneous flow of gas through them.

SPIROMETRY

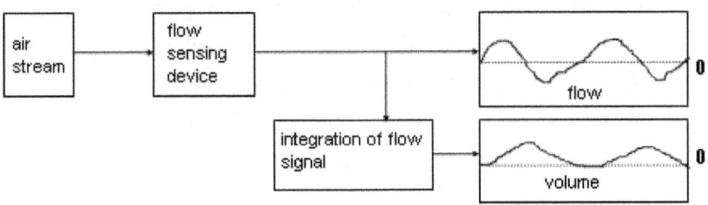

Figure 1-3. Diagram showing the steps followed to obtain the volume and flow signals with a flow-sensing device.

The most commonly applied principle is the differential pressure flow, in which the pressure drop across a slight resistance placed in the stream is proportional to the flow of gas. A very low pressure difference (usually less than 2 cm H_2O) is created when air flows through the device. A simplified mathematical expression relating the difference in pressure between the two ends of the tube, the flow and the resistance of the tube can be written as follows:

Pressure difference = resistance x flow   equation 1

If the composition of the gas passing through the tube does not change, the flow is laminar, and the resistance in the tube is constant, then we have:

Pressure difference = K x flow   equation 2

In equation 2, K is a constant value. Therefore, under the conditions described above, measurement of the pressure difference between the two ends of the tube is a proportional measurement of the flow of gas through the device. Measurement of the pressure difference is usually made by an electronic differential pressure transducer that rapidly measures the pressure when airflow also changes rapidly, as during breathing maneuvers (Figure 1-4).

The Fleisch pneumotachograph is the oldest, and probably the most frequently used device in this type of spirometers. It consists of a bundle of capillary tubes that provide a small fixed resistance to airflow (Figure 1-4). The same principle applies to the screen pneumotachographs (Lilly type pneumotachometers) where a fine mesh-screen is the flow resistor element.

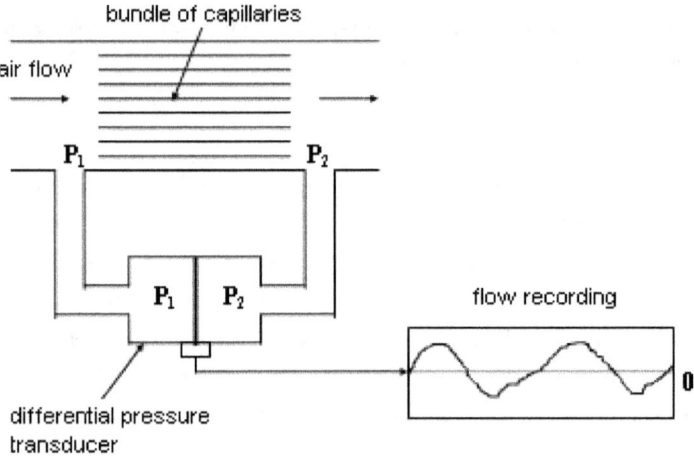

Figure 1-4. Diagram of the measurement of flow with a Fleisch pneumotachograph.

Modern electronic spirometers not only measure and calculate volume and/or flow, according to the measuring device, but also automatically make the necessary data corrections to make it possible to compare results obtained in different ambient conditions and in different laboratories.

Gas volume in the lungs is at body temperature and atmospheric pressure and is completely saturated with water vapor at body temperature. These conditions are commonly abbreviated BTPS (Body Temperature Pressure Saturated). If the sensing device is heated and located close to the patient's mouth, the exhaled air will still be at about body temperature and 100 % humidity, and no BTPS correction will be necessary for the measurement. However, if the volume or flow sensing device is located at the end of a long length of tubing, the exhaled air will cool down toward room (ambient) temperature before it passes through or into the device. Under these conditions, the gas is still saturated with water vapor, but the water vapor volume is reduced at the lower temperature. These conditions are abbreviated ATPS (Ambient Temperature Pressure Saturated). It means that under given laboratory conditions (ATPS), the actual lung volume (BTPS) will shrink, in response to the ambient temperature as long as it is lower than body temperature, and the observed ATPS volumes must therefore be corrected back to conditions prevailing in the lungs. Calculation of corrected data is made by computerized spirometers, according to the ambient temperature and barometric pressure measured by the machine or previously entered manually and stored in the memory of the machine (See Appendix for description of the calculations). In the case of flow-sensing devices, appropriate corrections vary according to the spirometer system, type and size of pneumotachographs.

José Almirall

Chapter 2

WHAT DO WE MEASURE WITH SPIROMETRY?

In general, to ventilate means to expose to a current of fresh, purifying or refreshing air. The main function of the respiratory system is to ventilate the lungs for keeping the process of gas exchange between the lungs and the blood working adequately. Spirometry is a pulmonary function test used to evaluate the process of pulmonary ventilation.

Pulmonary ventilation

The respiratory tract is composed of a series of branching tubes that form the conducting airways up to the terminal bronchioles which are the smallest airways without alveoli. Then branching continues in the terminal lung units (acini) which are the parts of lungs distal to the terminal bronchioles, i.e. respiratory bronchioles, alveolar ducts, alveolar sacs and alveoli. Pulmonary ventilation is the cyclic process of the movement of the inspired air through the upper air passages and subdivisions of the conducting airways into the terminal respiratory units, and from the latter back to outside the body. Part of the fresh air entering the respiratory system during each inspiration reaches the alveoli of the acini where exchange of gases with the blood occurs, thus producing the alveolar ventilation. The other part is merely moved in and out of the conducting airways. As conducting airways are not anatomically capable of exchanging gas with the blood, the space within them (about 150 ml) is called the anatomical dead space.

Branching airways become narrower, shorter, and more numerous as they penetrate deeper into the lungs. Although the resulting branches are smaller than the parent stem, their total cross section is always greater, so that the total cross sectional area increases from trachea to alveolar sacs. The increase in total cross sectional area is extremely rapid in the terminal respiratory units as compared to conducting airways (Figure 2-1), and has important implications in the way air is moved into the lungs during inspiration.

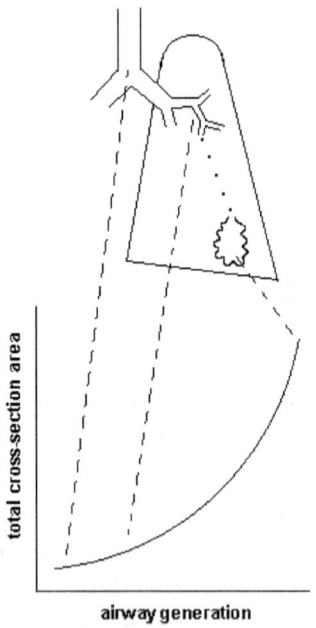

Figure 2-1. Change in cross-sectional area in the bronchial tree as a function of airway generation.

The air is drawn into the lungs by the increase in volume brought about by contraction of the inspiratory muscles, and it flows through the large airways down to about the terminal bronchioles by bulk flow, like water through a pipe. Upon entry of inspired air into the respiratory units, the increase of cross sectional area is so large that the forward velocity of the gas becomes very small, like smoke that flows through pursed lips into a big room. Under those conditions, diffusion becomes the main determinant of gas distribution within the respiratory zone, where gas-flow rates are minimal and diffusion distances are very small. In a few words, mass movement or bulk flow is principally of importance in the large airways, whereas diffusion of gas takes over as the dominant mechanism of ventilation in the small lung units.

Differences in the dominant mechanism of ventilation in the airways have influence on the resistance to airflow. Most of the resistance to airflow is in the upper and large central airways, whereas peripheral airway resistance (airway smaller than 2-3 mm diameter) is small.[3] These observations about the partitioning of trachea-bronchial resistance have important implications with regard to disease. The peripheral airways are the site of obstruction in a variety of diseases, the most important of which are chronic bronchitis and emphysema. Because these airways contribute very little to total flow resistance, significant disease may occur in them before measurements of pulmonary resistance or spirometry tests will detect obstruction. For this reason the peripheral airways have been called the "quiet zone" of the lung, and this has led to a search for tests and methods for identifying early obstruction in small airways before diseases are far advanced.

Pulmonary ventilation is not uniformly distributed in all regions of the lungs. Due to the effect of gravity, there is a gradient of intrapleural pressure which is more negative in the uppermost regions and less negative in the lowermost regions. The pressure gradient from top to bottom is larger in the upright position than in the supine position. This way, in the resting end-expiratory position of the lungs, alveoli in the top regions of the lungs are exposed to a more negative pressure and are more expanded than alveoli in the bottom regions. When inspiratory muscles contract and expand the thoracic cage and the lungs, the change in volume in the bottom regions (less expanded at the beginning of inspiration) can be larger than in the top regions (already more expanded at the beginning of inspiration). In other words, the bottom regions of the lungs receive a larger part of the inspired air volume and are more ventilated than the top regions. This unequal distribution of the inspired air in the lungs is called regional ventilation. In a normal situation, the lowermost regions in the lungs also receive a larger proportion of the lung blood perfusion than the uppermost regions. Therefore, normally, there is a good match between the amount of ventilation and perfusion arriving to the different regions, i.e. there is a good ventilation-perfusion relationship and thus a good blood oxygenation. In pathologic conditions, a ventilation-perfusion mismatch may occur and lead to impaired blood oxygenation.

Limitations of spirometry

Spirometry is a physiologic test that can only indicate how disease has altered the ventilatory function. Many factors may contribute to the development of ventilatory impairment. Spirometry tests do not reveal alterations in all types of pulmonary disease but only in those that disturb the ventilatory function sufficiently to recognize with certainty the deviation from normal values. Measurements made with spirometry are limited to the ventilatory aspect of respiration in general. With spirometry, we cannot have information about the regional ventilation nor can we detect whether there is a ventilation-perfusion mismatch.

The main function of the lungs is to ventilate the blood. Mechanisms to adjust minute ventilation or to relate perfusion to ventilation within the lungs may be so efficient, that gas tensions in blood may remain within normal limits despite the presence of extensive lung disease or marked changes in respiratory mechanics. It is very important to understand that no single test of lung function can ever measure all the attributes that constitute its totality. As mentioned before, spirometry can only indicate alterations in the ventilatory function. Spirometry may be normal, but other tests may show that other aspects of the respiratory function (e.g. gas exchange) are impaired.

The physiological factors influencing the ventilatory function are dependent on the overall mechanical properties of the lungs. For this reason, although spirometry is used to measure directly the ventilatory function of the lungs, it also provides information that allows drawing some indirect conclusions about the interaction of forces and resistance to accomplish ventilation, i.e. the respiratory mechanics. For example, the decrease in vital capacity in patients with pulmonary fibrosis that can be detected with spirometry may be interpreted as an increase in the resistance opposing to the expansion of the lungs but this resistance is not directly measured by spirometry.

Spirometry tests

We can measure the volume of inspired and/or expired gas with spirometry, but we cannot measure the volume of gas remaining in the lungs after a complete expiration. Measurement of the volume of gas entering or leaving the lungs is what spirometry tests are all about. In our days, the test of forced expiration is the symbol of spirometry. However there are other spirometry tests that also provide useful information.

Static lung volumes

Subdivisions of lung volume are recorded by having the subject breathe through a spirometer that provides a volume-time spirogram. The maneuvers to measure lung volume subdivisions are usually slow, and both begin and end in static or nearly static efforts. For that reason lung volume subdivisions are frequently called static volumes (Figure 2-2). Like other lung volumes, they are usually reported in terms of BTPS (see Appendix).

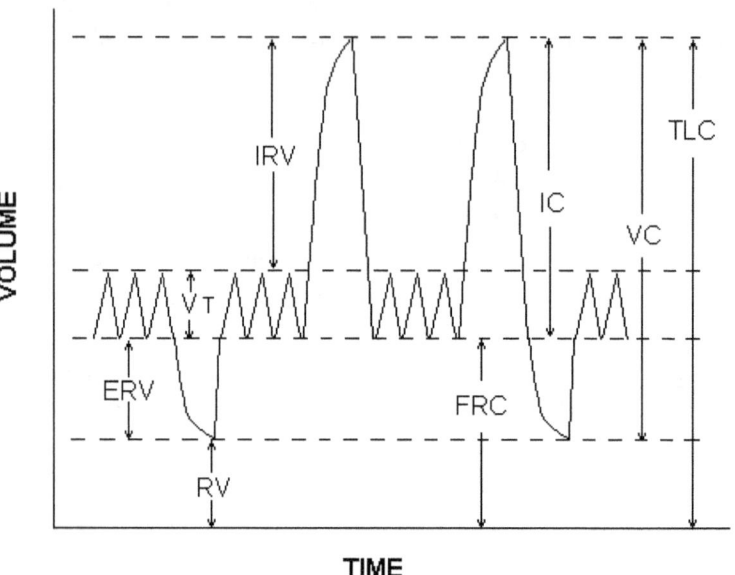

Figure 2-2. Schematic representation of a spirogram with the various subdivisions of the lung volume. VT = tidal volume; ERV = expiratory reserve volume; IRV = inspiratory reserve volume; RV = residual volume; FRC = functional residual capacity; IC = inspiratory capacity; VC = vital capacity; TLC = total lung capacity.

The subdivisions of the lung volume that can be measured by spirometry are the following:

- Tidal volume (V_T, TV is also used): volume of air inhaled or exhaled with each breath during normal breathing.
- Inspiratory reserve volume (IRV): maximal volume of air inhaled from the end-inspiratory level of the tidal volume.

- Expiratory reserve volume (ERV): maximal volume of air exhaled from the end-expiratory level of the tidal volume.

Combinations of lung volumes are referred as to lung capacities:

- Inspiratory capacity (IC): the sum of IRV and V_T (maximal volume of air that can be inspired beginning from the end-expiratory level of the tidal volume).
- Vital capacity (VC): maximal volume of air exhaled from the point of maximum inspiration, encompassing IRV, V_T, and ERV. The symbol IVC should be used for the inspiratory vital capacity; which is the maximal volume of air inhaled from the point of maximum expiration.

The lung volume subdivisions and lung capacities mentioned above can be measured with many spirometers used in clinical settings, but the measurements are frequently used only for research. For example, the measurement of the inspiratory capacity (IC) has been used as an expression of hyperinflation in chronic obstructive pulmonary disease (COPD).[4]

The IC has also been found to be sensitive and reliable for assessing therapeutic responses.[5]

Lung volume subdivision and pulmonary capacities that include the volume of air trapped in the lungs after a maximal expiratory effort cannot be measured by spirometry alone. They are the following (Figure 2-2):

- Residual volume (RV): volume of air remaining in the lungs after maximal exhalation.
- Functional residual capacity (FRC): the sum of RV and ERV, volume of air remaining in the lungs at end-expiratory position of the tidal volume.

- Total lung capacity (TLC): the sum of all volume compartments or the volume of air in the lungs after maximal inspiration.

Measurement of these lung volumes can be made using different special methods such as body plesthysmography, nitrogen washout from the lungs, inert gas dilution, and imaging techniques which allow estimating the volume of air trapped in the lungs after a complete expiration. Details of such methods are out of the scope of this book.

Minute ventilation

The minute ventilation or pulmonary ventilation per minute is the total volume of air that enters and leaves the lungs each minute. The units are usually ml/min or L/min. Minute ventilation can be expressed either as expiratory ($\dot{V}_E$) or inspiratory ($\dot{V}_I$). Indeed, more O_2 is absorbed from the alveoli than CO_2 is added in such a way that normally there is a difference of about 50 ml/min between the O_2 uptake and the CO_2 elimination. Therefore, the inspired ventilation per minute ($\dot{V}_I$) is slightly larger than the expired ventilation ($\dot{V}_E$), but for simplicity they are considered as equals.

Minute ventilation can be calculated from a spirogram by adding the measured tidal volume (V_T) of each breath during a minute, but actually that is not a usual way of calculating it. The average minute ventilation calculated from three or four consecutive breaths in a spirogram is more appropriately used for representing the events during a minute. Minute ventilation can be expressed by the equation $\dot{V}_E = V_T \times f$, where f is frequency of breathing. In steady state, $\dot{V}_E$ can be calculated from a single breath by dividing V_T by the total duration of a breathing cycle, T_{Tot} ($f = 1/T_{Tot}$) (Figure 2-3). It should be noted that if T_{Tot} is measured in seconds, and f is expressed in breathings per min, then $f = 60/T_{Tot}$.

Pulmonary ventilation per minute can be calculated from the

volume and frequency components of a complete tidal breathing cycle, but there is another way of expressing the breathing cycle.[6] If we consider $\overset{\bullet}{V}_I$, it follows that

$$\overset{\bullet}{V}_I = (V_T/T_I) \times (T_I/T_{Tot})$$

where T_I is inspiratory time and V_T/T_I is the mean inspiratory flow rate; T_{tot} is the total respiratory cycle duration and T_I/T_{Tot} represents the fraction of inspiration duration (also called duty cycle, or the fraction of the breathing cycle in which inspiratory muscles are "on duty").

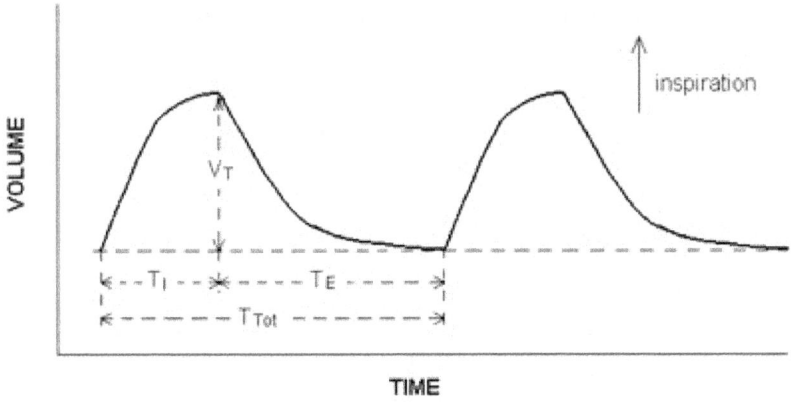

Figure 2-3. Recording of quiet breathing.

Expressing $\overset{\bullet}{V}_I$ as a function of V_T/T_I and T_I/T_{Tot} provides additional information. In man, the inspiratory volume-time profile is usually approximately linear.[6] Therefore, if inspiration starts at FRC and the mechanical properties of the respiratory system do not change, the V_T/T_I reflects the 'inspiratory drive'. In other words, under such conditions V_T/T_I is an index of the neural output of the respiratory centers to the inspiratory muscles.

Measurements of tidal volume and resting minute ventilation are rarely made in office pulmonary assessment since patients with advanced lung disease usually have resting ventilation with normal tidal volume and respiratory rate. In addition, when patients know that their ventilation is being measured, they pay more attention to their breathing, and the breathing pattern may be altered. The presence of the nose clip and the mouthpiece may also contribute to change the rate and depth of breathing. However, these aspects of pulmonary ventilation have been very helpful to study the physiopathology of some pulmonary conditions. For example, it has been observed that patients with chronic obstructive pulmonary disease (COPD) and high concentration of carbon dioxide in blood (hypercapnia) maintain resting minute ventilation at a level that is below the one at which they could attain a normal concentration of carbon dioxide in blood, i.e. they maintain a state of hypoventilation.[7] This has made minute ventilation and its mechanisms of control important aspects of research efforts on COPD.

Maximal voluntary ventilation

The maximal voluntary ventilation (MVV) is the volume of gas that can be breathed per minute during maximal voluntary hyperventilation. In the test, the patient is instructed to breathe as deeply and as rapidly as he can; he is encouraged to imitate the type of breathing used during severe exercise choosing his own frequency and tidal volume. The test is usually continued for 10 or 15 seconds and the gas volume is corrected to liters per minute (Figure 2-4).

Considerable coaching and some practice are required for adequate performance of this test, and the 'learning effect' may cause some increments between first and second effort. A disadvantage of this test is that its performance requires the maximal respiratory muscular effort of which the patient is capable, and a desire to cooperate even to the point of exhaustion. Not every patient is motivated to this extent.

SPIROMETRY

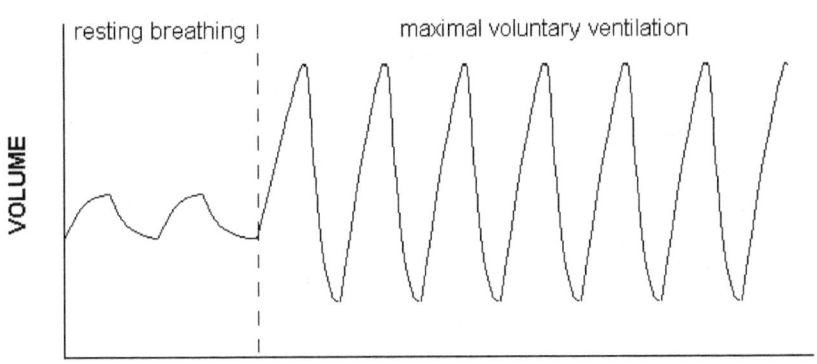

Figure 2-4. Spirogram illustrating the recorded MVV in a normal subject.

The MVV is affected by factors such as the muscular force available, the compliance of the lungs and chest wall, and the resistance of the airways and lung and chest wall tissues. Thus, the MVV test gives information regarding the mechanics of breathing although, as any other pulmonary function test, a low value is not diagnostic of any single disease. Because of the large standard deviation observed in measurements of MVV, the normal range may include deviations of 25-35 % from mean group values. Inspection of the spirogram is of diagnostic value to observe occurrence of progressive trapping of air in patients with obstructive lung diseases.

Historically, the MVV preceded the test of forced expiration, but the former has been replaced by the latter because is simpler, less fatiguing, easily repeatable and clearly separate inspiratory and expiratory difficulties. Nevertheless, the MVV continues to be useful as an adjunct to noninvasive cardiopulmonary exercise testing. Comparison of peak ventilation at exercise to the MVV permits computation of ventilatory reserve for a patient.

Forced expiration

The simplest maneuver to test lung function is a forced expiration. In the test, the subject inspires to his/her maximal lung volume, then blows out as forcefully as possible, and keeps expiring to as low a lung volume as possible. The volume of the forced expiration starting at the full inspiratory position is measured in relation to time. Figure 2-5 shows a forced expiratory maneuver in a volume-time spirogram. There are spirometers in which the graphic representation of the forced expiratory maneuver shows exhaled volume going downwards in a volume-time spirogram, as in Figure 2-5. There are other spirometers in which the graphical representation of exhaled volume goes upwards.

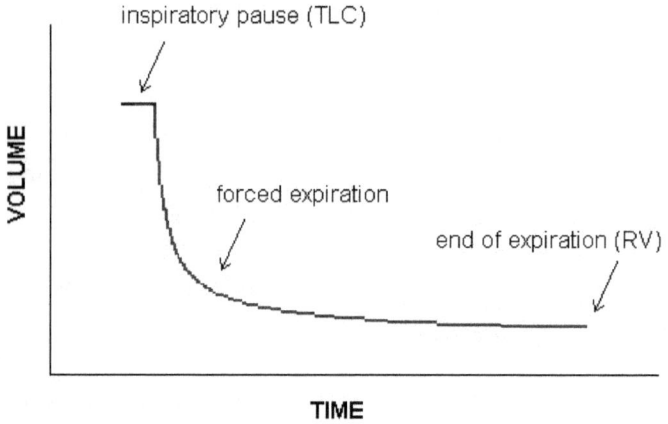

Figure 2-5. Volume-time curve of the forced expiratory maneuver.

The volume-time spirogram of the forced expiratory maneuver showing the maximal rate at which air is exhaled is called the forced vital capacity (FVC) curve (Figure 2-5). However, the maximal flow rate of the exhaled air can also be measured and the instantaneous expiratory flow at different lung volumes can be recorded, as from a flow-volume curve. This way, we can obtain the maximal expiratory flow-volume curve (MEFV) which is another way of recording the forced expiratory maneuver (Figure 2-6).

In the normal MEFV curve, flow increases rapidly, reaches a maximum at about 80 % of the vital capacity (i.e. after 20 % of the vital capacity is exhaled), and then decreases, reaching a value of zero at residual volume (Figure 2-6). In fact, the MEFV curve contains essentially the same information as the FVC curve, and can be derived from it.

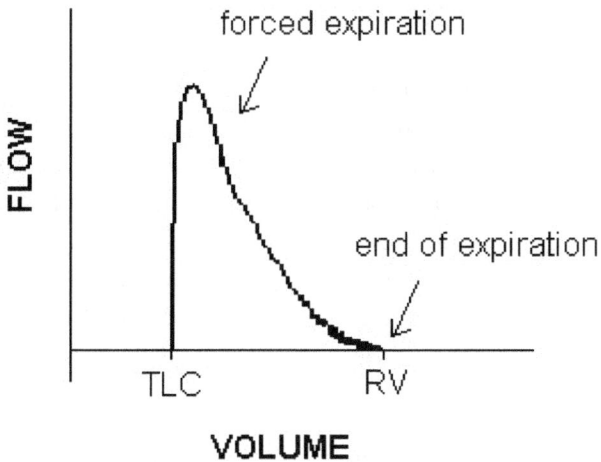

Figure 2-6. Flow-volume curve of the forced expiratory maneuver or maximal expiratory flow-volume curve (MEFV). TLC = total lung capacity, RV = residual volume.

However, flow is a noisy signal, with oscillations of physiological origin. Furthermore, relatively small differences in TLC decrease the reproducibility of successive MEFV curves. Nevertheless, recording of the MEFV curve is useful because it permits easier recognition of some abnormalities that produce characteristic patterns of the curve (see Chapter 5).

During a forced expiration, there is an effort-dependent portion above about 75 - 80 % of the total exhaled volume (first part of the expiration), and an effort-independent portion below 75 - 80 % of that volume. No defined limit to expiratory flow exists at volumes near to maximal lung inflation. The effort-dependent portion depends upon how rapidly the expiratory muscles can contract and is an expression of the force-velocity relationship of these muscles. The maximal flow (or peak flow) in this portion depends on how rapidly pleural pressure can be increased at the beginning of the forced expiration.

The effort-independent part of the MEFV shows the relationship between lung volume and the maximal expiratory flow that is possible at each volume. Beyond the point in which flow becomes effort independent, the maximum flow depends on lung volume in a way that it decreases more or less linearly with decreasing lung volume. Once enough effort has been used to reach this point, flow becomes limited at its maximal value, and increasing degrees of effort will not produce any further increase in flow.

Maximal expiratory flow limitation results from dynamic compression of the compliant airways. Pleural pressure is usually negative in sign (sub-atmospheric) during normal breathing but becomes considerably greater than atmospheric during forced expiration. Flow limitation depends upon changes in intra-thoracic pressures during forced expiration.

The phenomenon of expiratory flow limitation may be explained as follows. Because the lungs have elastic recoil, alveolar pressure is greater than pleural pressure at any moment during the forced expiratory maneuver. However, pressure in the mouth is zero. Thus, pressure inside the airways must be dissipated from alveolus to mouth. It follows that there must be a point or points somewhere along the intra-thoracic airways at which the pressure inside must be exactly equal to pleural pressure. Such points are called equal pressure points (EPP). As the pressure difference across the wall is zero at the site of the EPP, the airways between EPP and the thoracic outlet become dynamically compressed. This increases their resistance, and for a given increase in expiratory effort (i.e. more positive pressure), the dynamic compression of the airways is such that the resistance increases proportionally to the pressure change. Thus, we have on one hand a greater pressure producing flow and on the other a greater resistance to flow. The result is that eventually a pleural pressure is reached above which expiratory flows becomes limited and independent of effort. If one makes a greater effort there is no increase in flow. At high lung volumes (i.e. near maximal lung inflation) dynamic compression of the airways does not occur, and flow varies with effort. Dynamic compression starts to happen after 20 - 30 per cent of air has been exhaled, and requires lower expiratory effort at lower lung volume.

In normal subjects maximal flow rates are never used during exhaustive exercise. They are only used during coughing. Therefore, the reserves of the ventilatory apparatus are such that ventilation does not limit our ability to exercise. This is not the case in disease. If lung recoil, airway resistance, and/or airway compliance are impaired then maximal expiratory flows are reduced. Under these conditions, the airways will decrease in caliber or even collapse when faced with an increase in pleural pressure that normally does not produce such effects. It means that some patients may be using maximal expiratory flow rates during quiet breathing at rest and/or at exercise, and there is very little reserve by which they can increase ventilation (see Chapter 5).

Forced inspiration

In the maneuver of forced inspiration, starting from the position of full expiration, the subject inspires forcefully to as high a lung volume as possible. Figure 2-7 shows a forced inspiratory maneuver made after a forced expiratory maneuver in a volume-time spirogram. The maximal inspiratory flow-volume (MIFV) curve is another way of recording the forced inspiratory maneuver (Figure 2-8).

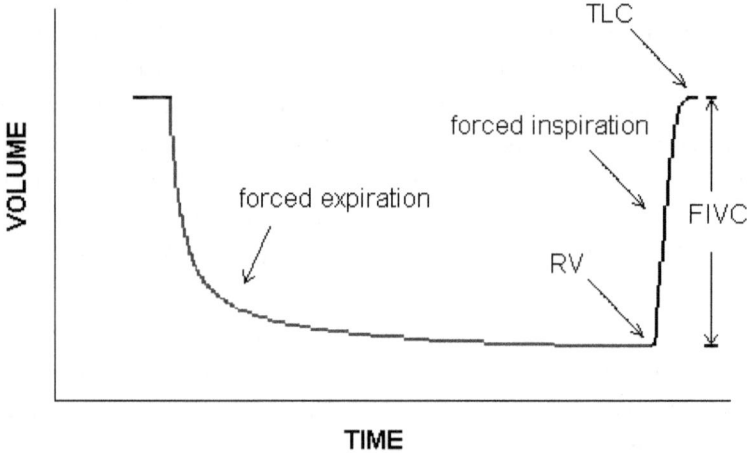

Figure 2-7. Volume-time curve of a forced expiratory maneuver followed by a forced inspiratory maneuver (RV = residual volume; TLC = total lung capacity; FIVC = forced inspiratory vital capacity).

The subject may reach the position of full expiration after a maneuver of forced expiration, as shown in Figure 2-7 and Figure 2-8. However, a full expiration can also be achieved after a slow expiration that started from functional residual capacity (FRC). It has been found that the ability of normal subjects to generate inspiratory flows at residual volume (RV) may change according to the type of expiratory maneuver preceding the forced inspiratory maneuver.[8] Up to date, standardization of lung function tests has not included recommendations for the forced inspiratory maneuver, and there is no universal agreement on the way to proceed. The 'best' forced inspiratory maneuver is not necessarily associated to the 'best' forced expiratory maneuver. Therefore, it has been suggested to obtain them separately, and then to display them together for a final evaluation.[8]

SPIROMETRY

The forced inspiratory maneuver is frequently made during spirometric testing, mostly if the flow-volume curve is used to monitor the test. However, the parameters derived from this maneuver are usually omitted in the results of the test, or they are not used in the elaboration of the final report.

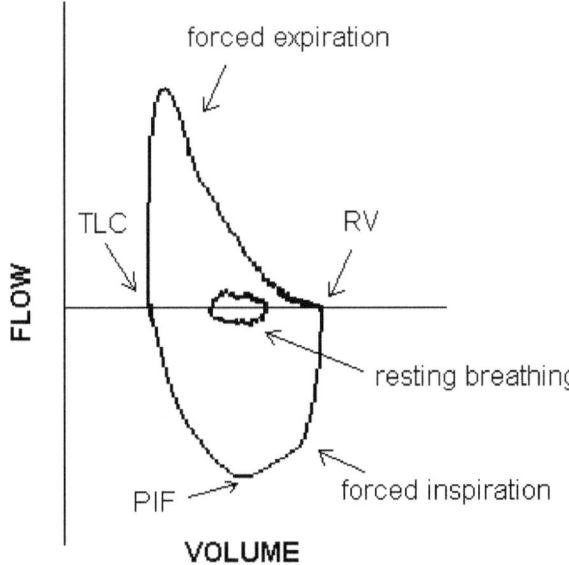

Figure 2-8. Diagram showing a MEFV curve followed by a MIFV curve (PIF = peak inspiratory flow, TLC= total lung capacity, RV = residual volume).

Use of the MIFV is often limited to obtain the record of a complete inspiratory-expiratory flow-volume curve, which may help to distinguish between intrathoracic and extrathoracic airways obstruction (see Chapter 5). A less common use of this maneuver is to differentiate expiratory flow limitation due to airways obstruction from that attributable solely to low elastic lung recoil from pulmonary emphysema, which would affect little the inspiratory flows.[9]

José Almirall

Chapter 3

FORCED EXPIRATION: PARAMETERS AND PERFORMANCE

A necessary step to make valid comparisons of different tests is to convert spirometry tests into measurable variables is. The description of parameters that follows does not intend to be exhaustive. Instead, only the most frequently used parameters are described.

Parameters measured from the forced expiratory volume-time curve

The simplest analysis of the forced expiratory spirogram is to measure the change in one variable (volume or time) for a fixed change in the other. Some common methods of quantifying the volume-time relationship of the forced expiratory maneuver are listed below.

Forced vital capacity (FVC)

The FVC is the volume of air expired after full inspiration, expiration being as rapid and complete as possible (Figure 3-1). It is usually measured in liters or milliliters.

The measurement of FVC in spirometry gives an idea of the volume contained in the lungs at the point of maximal inspiration. The ideal situation is to know the total lung capacity (TLC, see static lung volumes, Chapter 2) of the subject. However, the TLC cannot be measured by spirometry alone, and in many patients spirometry is the only pulmonary function test performed. Therefore, restrictive pulmonary defects (characterized by decreased TLC) are often inferred from the spirogram on the basis of a reduced FVC, or a reduced vital capacity (VC) if static lung volumes are measured.

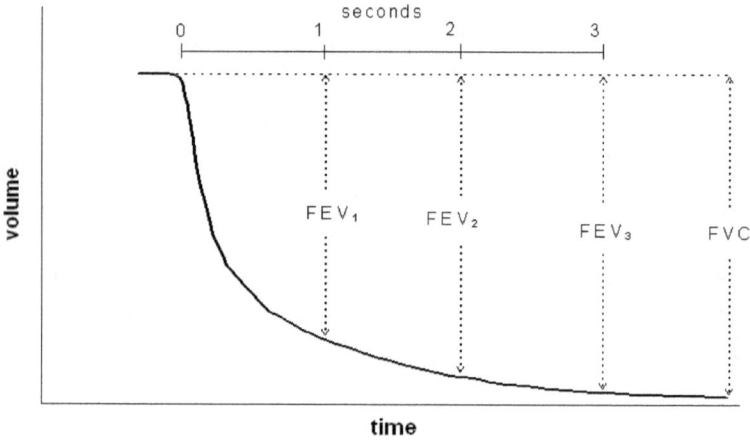

Figure 3-1. Measurement of some parameters from the forced expiratory volume-time curve.

In normal subjects, FVC and VC values are usually similar, and measuring only FVC gives a reliable value of the subject's vital capacity. In patients with obstructive diseases, measurements of both VC and FVC should be performed for the reasons explained in the following lines. Dynamic compression of the airways and expiratory flow limitation (see Chapter 2) may be enhanced because of the obstruction produced by either loss of elastic recoil or destruction of the peribronchiolar support, or due to the thickening of the airway wall and narrowing of the airway lumen by a chronic inflammatory process. In these cases, measurement of VC with slow maneuvers that both begin and end in nearly static efforts sometimes yields values of vital capacity dramatically higher than those of FVC in a way that a reduced FVC observed during forced expiration may no longer be appreciated after slow VC maneuvers. As a general rule, a normal value of FVC usually rules out the need to measure VC, but an abnormal value of FVC should always be accompanied by measurement of VC.

Forced expiratory volume in time interval t (FEVt)

It is the volume of air exhaled in the specified time during the performance of the forced vital capacity. It is measured in liters or milliliters. The forced expiratory volume can be measured over several periods of time, for example 0.75, 1, 2, 3, and 6 sec.; the results are given as $FEV_{0.75}$, FEV_1, FEV_2, etc. (Figure 3-1).

Forced expiratory volume in one second (FEV_1): The volume of air exhaled in the first second during the performance of the forced expiratory maneuver. The FEV_1 is considered the "gold standard" for pulmonary function tests since it generally relates well to the development and presence of clinical lung disease. It is the single most reproducible parameter of lung function test. Due to its low within-subject variability FEV_1 has been considered to have a better sensitivity to detect changes in airflow resistance than other indices that may be derived from the spirogram.

The FEV_1 is the most widely used parameter that reflects the resistance to airflow within the airways. However, the absolute value of FEV_1 has the limitation that reduced values may be observed when the total lung capacity is low (restrictive abnormality), without the presence of airway obstruction. This is the justification to calculate FEV_1 as a fraction of FVC (FEV_1/FVC).

The FEV_6 is the expiratory volume exhaled at 6 seconds during the performance of the forced expiratory maneuver. The FEV_6 was proposed as a surrogate for FVC and has been recommended for chronic obstructive pulmonary disease (COPD) screening. Frequently, patients with significant airway obstruction or elderly subjects need exhalation times longer than 6 seconds to reach a plateau during the forced expiratory maneuver. The advantage of stopping the expiratory maneuver after 6 seconds is to decrease the physical demands of performing the maneuver. Multiple prolonged exhalations may cause discomfort and exhalations longer than 6 seconds are not justified in many cases. However, some limitations to the use of FEV_6 for detecting airway obstruction have been reported.[10-13]

It should be noted that the largest observed volume during the first 6 seconds of a forced expiratory maneuver was named FVC_6,[14] which is sometimes slightly bigger than the FEV_6. The small difference between FVC_6 and FEV_6 arises sometimes when the volume in the volume-time curve of the forced vital capacity maneuver slightly decreases immediately before the 6 s point. In such cases, the largest volume during the first 6 seconds of the maneuver (FVC_6) is really observed just before the curve reached the 6 seconds (FEV_6). For the sake of simplicity, the FEV_6 and the FVC_6 can be considered as equals.

Forced expiratory flow between 25% and 75% of the forced vital capacity ($FEF_{25-75\%}$)

The $FEF_{25-75\%}$ is the mean forced expiratory flow during the middle half of the FVC, i.e. the mean flow measured in the two medial quarters of the FVC. It was formerly called the maximum mid-expiratory flow rate (MMFR) (Figure 3-2). It is measured in liters/s.

The value of $FEF_{25-75\%}$ as spirometry index of airway obstruction is a controversial issue. Some authors consider $FEF_{25-75\%}$ a redundant parameter and do not use it, whereas others use it as a sensitive indicator of airflow obstruction. For example, it was reported that in asthmatic children with normal FEV_1, a low $FEF_{25-75\%}$ is associated with increased asthma severity, systemic steroid use, and asthma exacerbations.[15]

According to our experience, depending on the age of the subject, both opinions about the value of $FEF_{25-75\%}$ as spirometry index of airway obstruction are right. In subjects up to about 60 years of age, lower limits of normal of this parameter are useful to identify low values, and the $FEF_{25-75\%}$ is a sensitive indicator of airway obstruction. In these subjects, a test may suggest the presence of airway obstruction when there is a borderline value of FEV_1/FVC and low $FEF_{25-75\%}$. However, in older subjects $FEF_{25-75\%}$ is not more sensitive than FEV_1/FVC to detect airway obstruction.[16] In older subjects, the calculated lower limits of normal for $FEF_{25-75\%}$ may be so low that may not detect abnormalities that are detected with FEV_1/FVC.

A criticism to the $FEF_{25-75\%}$ has been that it is greatly affected by the absolute volume at which measurement is made, and therefore, the size of the FVC. During forced expiration, even cooperative subjects may change the starting volume or expired volume in different efforts yielding different values of $FEF_{25-75\%}$. Nevertheless, it is generally accepted that if the FEV_1/FVC ratio is borderline, normal values of $FEF_{25-75\%}$ may be taken into account to rule out obstruction from a spirogram.

Abnormal values of $FEF_{25-75\%}$ have been considered to have low specificity to diagnose obstruction.[17] However, our experience is that this limitation only seems to apply when this parameter is used as an index of airway obstruction in subjects with low FVC, which is something that should not be done. When FVC is low, $FEF_{25-75\%}$ is not a good index of airway obstruction.

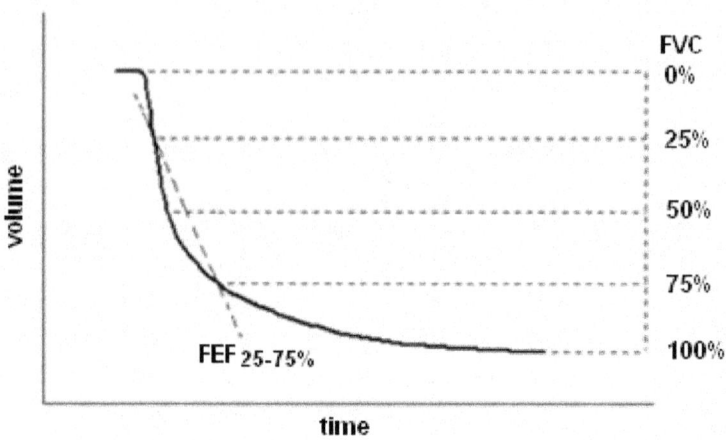

Figure 3-2. Measurement of FEF25-75% from the forced expiratory volume-time curve.

As occurs with FEV_1, the absolute value of $FEF_{25-75\%}$ has the limitation that it may be reduced without the presence of airway obstruction when the total lung capacity (and hence, FVC) is low. When FVC is within normal limits (and the total lung capacity is also normal), abnormal values of $FEF_{25-75\%}$ are indicative of airway obstruction.

The forced expiratory flow between 25% and 75% of the largest observed volume during the first 6 seconds of a forced vital capacity maneuver ($FEF_{25-75\%6}$) is the mean forced expiratory flow during the middle half of the expired volume of a maneuver stopped at 6s. This parameter should be measured when the FEV_6 is used as surrogate for FVC.

Forced expiratory volume (timed) to forced vital capacity ratio (FEVt/FVC)

The most widely used is the forced expiratory volume in one second to forced vital capacity ratio (FEV$_1$/FVC), expressed as a fraction or a percentage.

The FEV$_1$/FVC ratio is considered the primary guide for distinguishing obstructive from non-obstructive spirometry patterns. It is generally accepted that a decreased FEV$_1$/FVC ratio is the expression of airflow limitation.

The forced expiratory volume in one second to forced expiratory volume in 6 seconds ratio (FEV$_1$/FEV$_6$), expressed as a fraction or a percentage can be calculated when FEV$_6$ is used as a surrogate for FVC. However, it has been reported that FEV$_1$/FEV$_6$ has lower sensitivity than FEV$_1$/FEV$_1$ for detecting airway obstruction.[10,12] The FEV$_1$/FEV$_6$ has been recommended as an additional parameter that may provide useful information in some patients, but should not be used for replacing the FEV$_1$/FEV$_1$ as the standard for airways obstruction.[13]

Parameters measured from the forced expiratory flow-volume curve

Some common methods of quantifying the flow-volume relationship of the forced expiratory maneuver are described here below.

Peak expiratory flow (PEF or PEFR)

It is the maximal value of flow (L/min or L/s) measured (Figure 3-3). The measurement of PEF is equivalent to a spot measurement of the slope of the FVC curve (volume vs. time) at its steepest point or the highest forced expiratory flow measured with a peak flow meter. This will occur in the upper half of the vital capacity, and is therefore influenced by the effort made during the early part of a forced expiration.

Forced expiratory flow related to some portion of the FVC curve (FEFx)

Modifiers refer to the amount of the FVC already exhaled when the measurement is made (Figure 3-3).

Instantaneous forced expiratory flow *after 25 %* of FVC *has been exhaled* (FEF25%)

Instantaneous forced expiratory flow *after 50 %* of FVC *has been exhaled* (FEF50%)

Instantaneous forced expiratory flow *after 75 %* of FVC *has been exhaled* (FEF75%)

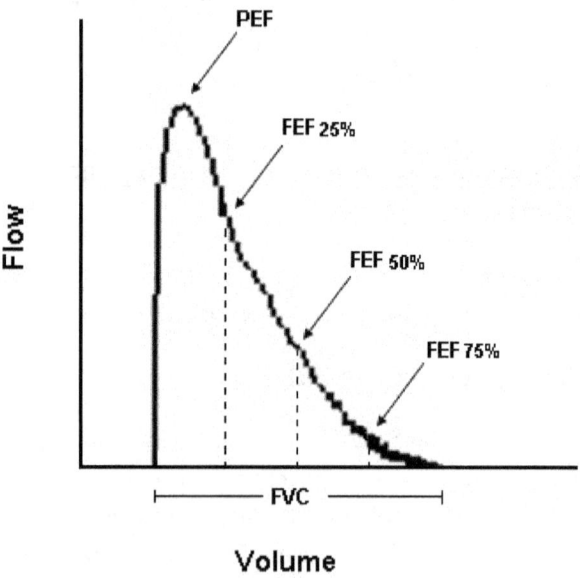

Figure 3-3. Measurement of parameters from the forced expiratory flow-volume curve.

Performance of the test of forced expiration

For results of the forced expiratory maneuver to be valid the test must be performed in a standardized manner. The American Thoracic Society (ATS) and the European Respiratory Society (ERS) have published guidelines to assist those performing spirometry tests.[2,18] Recommendations include equipment performance, validation and quality control, subject performance, and measurement procedures to determine acceptability and reproducibility. A detailed description of all these recommendations is out of the scope of this work. Only a brief description is presented below.

The test can be carry out in the sitting position or standing up. In the sitting position, the mouthpiece should be slightly elevated in order to have the neck in extension. In sitting or upright position, the test is done, if possible, with a nose clip. The subject must loosen any element being able to block his/her breathing, like a collar or a belt. The mouthpiece must be held firmly in the mouth. It is necessary to explain to the patient that he/she must firmly tighten the mouthpiece with the lips to avoid any escape of air responsible of error.

Spirometry depends upon the effort, cooperation and instruction of the subject performing the test. The cooperation of the patient is essential. The person administrating the test should relax the patient, explain the goal of the test and the maneuvers, and then stimulate the patient with the voice and gestures to obtain the best possible values. A learning effect is expected to lead to larger test values. On the contrary, decreasing motivation leads to lower values.

During the forced expiratory maneuver, subjects should exert maximal effort from the beginning. Spirometry maneuvers identified as showing an initial sub maximal effort should be discarded. This can be assessed using peak expiratory flow rate as an index of effort.

Recommended acceptability criteria on performing the test of forced expiration are the following:

1) Satisfactory start of the test: the maneuver should start with a fast maximal effort.

2) Spirogram free from artifacts: continuous blow as fast and as hard as possible, without cough, variable effort, early termination, etc.

3) A satisfactory exhalation: exhalation time of 6 seconds and/or plateau in the volume-time-curve; or reasonable duration or a plateau.

The acceptability criteria must be applied before the reproducibility criteria. Unacceptable maneuvers should be discarded before applying the reproducibility criteria. However, failure to meet acceptability criteria does not mean that the maneuver is useless.

We may have in front of us the results of a spirometry test in which the 'best' maneuver is not completely acceptable. In this cases, we should keep in mind a wise recommendation made by the American Thoracic Society on standardization of spirometry.[19]

> "...it cannot be overemphasized that failure to meet these criteria does not necessarily invalidate the maneuver, since for some subjects this is their best performance. Furthermore, such maneuvers should be retained, since these maneuvers may contain useful information."

Less than two acceptable forced expiratory maneuvers is a criterion for unacceptable subject performance. In these cases, just reporting values of FVC and FEV1 that at least the subject achieved could be useful information. Studies using spirometric lung function should take into account subjects who have exhibited test failure because exclusion of these subjects could be a source of bias in the results.

There are some subjects, mostly elderly, with normal lung function who are unable to meet the recommended end-of-test criteria.[2] This inability may merely reflect that these subjects are not willing to exhale longer.[20] However, acceptability and reproducibility criteria may also be difficult to satisfy for certain patients. Test failures have been associated with higher prevalence of respiratory symptoms [21], lower levels of lung function, [22] bronchial hyper responsiveness to metacholine, and to smoking.[23] Therefore, test failures may by themselves be an indicator of respiratory illness.[23]

The reproducibility criteria are used as a guide to whether more than three acceptable FVC maneuvers are needed. The following reproducibility criteria are applied after three acceptable spirograms have been obtained:

1) The largest FVC and second largest FVC from acceptable curves are within 0.150 L of each other.

2) The largest FEV1 and the second largest FEV1 are within 0.150 L of each other.

3) If criteria 1 and 2 are not met, testing should be continued. Eight maneuvers are considered a practical upper limit for most subjects.

No spirogram should be rejected only because of its poor reproducibility, provided three acceptable maneuvers are obtained. In these cases, reproducibility of the test should be considered at the time of interpretation (e.g. the FVC maneuver may have triggered a bronchospasm that prevented reproducibility).

Exclusion spirometry

Availability of small portable spirometers has made possible that spirometry tests can be conducted not only in diagnostic laboratories of hospital settings, but also in physicians' offices, and even at patients' homes. Theoretically, lung ventilation could be assessed during individual patient interactions as part of the physical examination. Such assessment would provide the physician objective information of the pulmonary ventilation that otherwise can only be guessed by auscultation and other indirect signs and symptoms. However, ongoing spirometry quality standards are difficult to bring into the daily routine of a physician's office.

Having in mind the idea that something is better than nothing, an attempt to have at least some objective information about lung ventilation was the initiative of performing "exclusion spirometry".[24]

In exclusion spirometry, acceptable and reproducible results would be sought. However, the goal of the test would be to try to reach values within normal limits, even if results do not reach quality standards. Normal results would be sufficient to exclude ventilatory impairment, except in asthma. Abnormal results would require further testing in a diagnostic spirometry laboratory. The aim of the initiative was to enhance the compliance of general practitioners to use spirometers for screening.

Test of forced expiration without spirometer

Spirometers may be unavailable in remote areas and third world countries. In the absence of a spirometer, the method of blowing out a flame (match or candle) may allow documenting objectively the ventilatory function of the lungs. This crude assessment of the ventilatory function has been the object of several publications. [25-28]

In the most recent publication,[25] the test was performed by holding a lightened candle perpendicular to a horizontal wooden board. The flame height was that of the subject's mouth and one edge of the board just touched the chest of the subject. After a maximum inspiration, the subjects attempted to blow the flame out with pursed lips. The farthest distance at which the subjects were able to extinguish the flame of the candle was recorded as 'candle distance'. The candle distance was best correlated with the forced expiratory volume in 1s (FEV1) ($r = 0.84$). The regression equation calculated was:

$$\text{FEV}_1 \text{ (L)} = 0.037659 \times \text{candle distance (cm)} + 0.4983$$

Estimated values of FEV$_1$ using the above regression are shown in Table 3-1.

Table 3-1. FEV1 estimated according to candle distance.

Candle distance (cm)	FEV1 (L)
15	1.06
20	1.25
25	1.44
30	1.63
35	1.82
40	2.00
45	2.19
50	2.38
55	2.57

José Almirall

Chapter 4

VARIABILITY IN SPIROMETRY

As a clinical test, spirometry is subject to technical variation, biologic variation, and variation produced by dysfunction or disease. Usually, the interest of clinicians is to discover any variation produced by dysfunction or disease. However, to do this, the variation caused by technical factors must be minimized and the biological variation has to be taken into account. In spirometry, the technical variation may be related not only to the instrument but also to the performance of subjects during the test and to the skills of the person administrating the test. Guidelines published by the American Thoracic Society and the European Respiratory Society on equipment performance, validation and quality control, subject performance, and measurement procedures are excellent references to minimize variation caused by technical factors.[2,18] The guidelines are of obligatory reading for those working with spirometers.

Once technical variability has been minimized, then biological variation has to be considered before attributing any observed variation to dysfunction or disease.

Biological variation

Intra-individual variability

Within-individual biological variation of spirometry results may be dependent on circadian rhythms (the lowest values in the early morning and the largest values around noon), body position (sitting, supine or standing), or head position (hyperextension or flexion of the neck). Therefore, uniformity in the time of testing and body position is necessary to avoid these sources of variation. Other possible biologic sources of variation in repeated spirometry tests are the environment (e.g. exposure to environmental pollutants), smoking, the intake of drugs, endocrine effects (e.g. menstrual cycle), and variability in the activity of a disease process (e.g. a cold or infection).

Inter-individual variability

Normal biologic sources of variability between individuals in spirometry results are sex, size, age and race.

Spirometric data of a subject can be evaluated by comparison with the distribution of measurements in a reference healthy population of similar anthropometric characteristics. Lung function increases with age during childhood and adolescence, and then declines. However, there is evidence indicating differences in the chronological age at which lung functions start to decline.

Regarding sex, males tend to outperform females with the same anthropometric characteristics. In each case, taller subjects have larger lung volume. In relation to race, controlling for sex, age, and standing height, when compared with Caucasians of European descent, other races usually show lower lung volume. Interracial differences in pulmonary function are partly due to differences in relative trunk height.

It has been hypothesized that the substantial disparity in

maximal expiratory flows among adults of similar lung volumes may reflect inter-individual differences in airway size relative to lung parenchyma size. This is called the dysanapsis hypothesis.[29] It means that individuals with large maximal expiratory flows for their lung volumes would have large airways in relation to their lung parenchyma size compared with the population as a whole, and vice versa. This inter-subject variability is present in early childhood and remains constant during growth.

Variation due to dysfunction or disease

Past and present health should be considered when evaluating lung function because lung function at a given moment of life reflects not only the present health but also all the damage the lung may have suffered in the past, starting from the prenatal period.

Ventilatory impairments that can be discovered by spirometry are essentially of two types, obstructive and restrictive abnormalities. Both ventilatory impairments may co-exist in the same subject and then it is said that there is a mixed abnormality.

Variation due to airway obstruction

Airway obstruction produces a decrease of maximal airflow from the lungs. However, a reduction of maximal airflow could be simply the result of a smaller lung volume. Therefore, an obstructive ventilatory defect is better defined as a disproportionate reduction of the maximal airflow with respect to the maximal lung volume, i.e. the total lung capacity. In spirometry, it is not possible to measure the total lung capacity, thus, maximal airflow from the lungs is compared to the maximal volume that can be displaced from the lungs, which is the vital capacity. The spirometry test is very useful to reveal an increased airway resistance due to airway obstruction.

Variation due to restriction of lung excursion

A restrictive defect is considered to be present when there is a reduction (or restriction) in the pulmonary expansion or excursion due to causes other than airflow obstruction. This is observed in lung resection and in clinical illnesses producing abnormalities of the lung parenchyma (e.g., fibrosis), chest wall (e.g., kyphoscoliosis), or respiratory muscles (e.g., dystrophies), i.e., abnormalities opposing to or impairing the normal expansion of the respiratory system during inspiration. The restrictive defect is suspected when measurements of lung volumes show a reduced vital capacity and there is no evidence of obstruction of airways. The presence of a restrictive defect is confirmed by a reduced total lung capacity. However, the total lung capacity cannot be measured by spirometry.

Variation due to a mixed abnormality

Obstructive and restrictive abnormalities may coexist in the same subject, but the way in which these two simultaneous processes affect the ventilatory function of the lungs is complex and depends on the underlying mechanism producing each abnormality. Two situations will be explained to illustrate the complexity of this situation.

There are two main mechanisms leading to a decrease in maximal expiratory flow rates: 1) airway narrowing (e.g., bronchoconstriction, inflammation of the airways); 2) loss of elastic recoil producing expiratory collapse of the peripheral airways (see Forced Expiration, Chapter 2). On the other hand, as mentioned in the preceding section, there are three main mechanisms restricting the lung excursion of the lungs: 1) abnormalities in the parenchyma (e.g. resection, fibrosis); 2) abnormalities in the chest wall (including the intra-pleural space); 3) abnormalities in the respiratory muscles.

In a subject with bronchial asthma and kyphoscoliosis, the

respiratory restriction lies in the chest wall (reduction in chest wall compliance) but the lung compliance is not affected. In this case, if there is an obstructive abnormality due to acute bronchoconstriction, it is not expected to be hidden by the restrictive abnormality in the chest wall and the effects of both abnormalities can be detected by spirometry.

A different situation occurs when pulmonary emphysema and pulmonary fibrosis coexist. In emphysema, the mechanism of the obstruction is the loss of elastic recoil, and expiratory collapse of the peripheral airways with a decrease of maximal airflow from the lungs. As a result, there is air trapping and lung hyperinflation. Pulmonary fibrosis characteristically leads to a restriction of lung excursion, with small lung volumes and increased expiratory flow rates resulting from a reduction in lung compliance. In other words, pulmonary emphysema and fibrosis both affect airway mechanics and produce opposing effects on expiratory flow rates and lung volume. One of the possible results of this interaction is that the effects of each separate disease on lung mechanics cancel each other and spirometry results could be normal.[30] This situation illustrates the point addressed in Chapter 2 about the limitations of spirometry. These patients usually present severe compromise of gas exchange that can be evidenced measuring the diffusing capacity of the lungs. [30]

José Almirall

PART 2

SPIROMETRY INTERPRETATION

Chapter 5

GENERAL ASPECTS OF SPIROMETRY INTERPRETATION

A definition of interpreting is to explain or tell the meaning of something or to present it in understandable terms. In the case of spirometry interpretation, what we do is to analyze numerical and graphical results of a spirometry test to arrive to a conclusion about the pulmonary function and then express the results of the analysis in words which convey a meaning about the functional status.

Spirometry results can be divided in two parts; one is the spirogram or graphic display of the tests, and the other part is represented by the numeric results of the parameters that have been measured. During a spirometry test, subjects are asked to perform several maneuvers (usually no less than three) to evaluate the reproducibility of the test maneuvers (see Chapter 3). In some electronic spirometers, only one spirogram is shown on the screen. In others, all the maneuvers retained by the operator of the spirometer are shown simultaneously on the screen for comparison. Usually, the measured parameters are calculated automatically from each maneuver. There are spirometers designed to show the numbers corresponding to the best maneuver at the end of the test. In other cases, the display of numeric results may include calculations from several maneuvers, highlighting the best one. Also, numeric results may include a selection of the best ones even if obtained from different maneuvers.

For interpretation of spirometry tests, both parts of the results should be considered, the graphic display of the test and the numeric results. However, before analyzing graphical and numerical results we should also make an evaluation on the quality of the tests and describe any important element that could be relevant for interpreting the test.

Graphic results

The shape of the volume-time curve is very useful to judge the quality of the maneuvers. It allows detecting some problems during the performance of the test such as slow starts of maneuvers, sub maximal expiratory efforts and maneuvers that have been finished prematurely (Figure 5-1).[19,31]

The shape of the flow-volume (F-V) curve is also a source of valuable information. It may help distinguishing between diffuse airway obstruction in the bronchial tree and a localized obstruction of the major airways.[32] A typical F-V pattern observed in patients with diffuse airway obstruction is shown in Figure 5-2 along with the pattern of F-V loop found in normal subjects.

In the obstructive as well as in the normal pattern, the expiratory limb is roughly triangular whereas the inspiratory limb is approximately semicircular. During expiration, flow rises sharply reaching its peak at a lung volume close to 80% of the vital capacity, and decreases at a lower rate after the peak (Figure 5-2). However, the area inside the F-V loop is considerably reduced in patients with diffuse airway obstruction as compared to normal. As obstruction increases, the area inside the loop decreases. The expiratory side of the loop is predominantly affected.

For some patients with severe chronic obstructive pulmonary disease (COPD), expiratory flows during quiet breathing are higher than the flows at the same lung volume on the maximal expiratory flow-volume curve, as shown in Figure 5-3. This phenomenon can usually be seen in patients with FEV1 smaller than about 1.2 L.[33] It is a reflection of the collapsibility of the airways in severe COPD patients and their compression by the positive pleural pressure produced by contraction of the expiratory muscles during the forced expiratory maneuver.

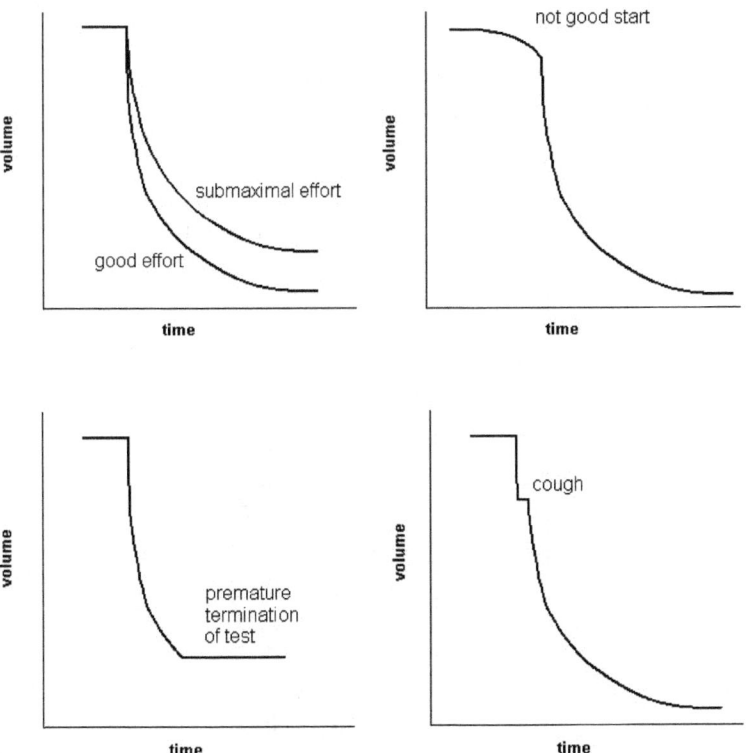

Figure 5-1. Some problems during the performance of the test of forced expiration as observed in the volume-time spirogram.

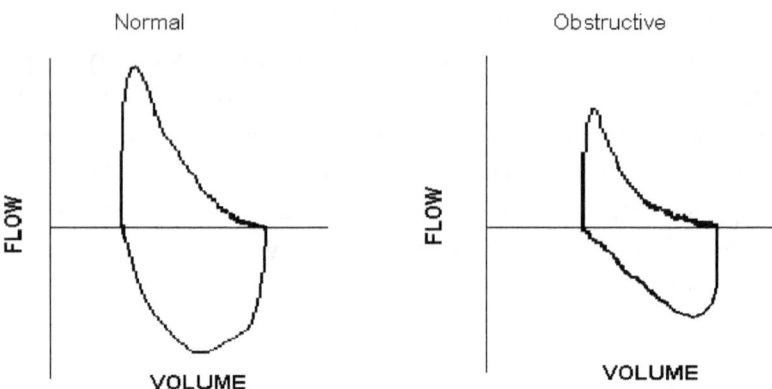

Figure 5-2. Characteristic flow-volume loops seen in normal subjects and in patients with diffuse airway obstruction.

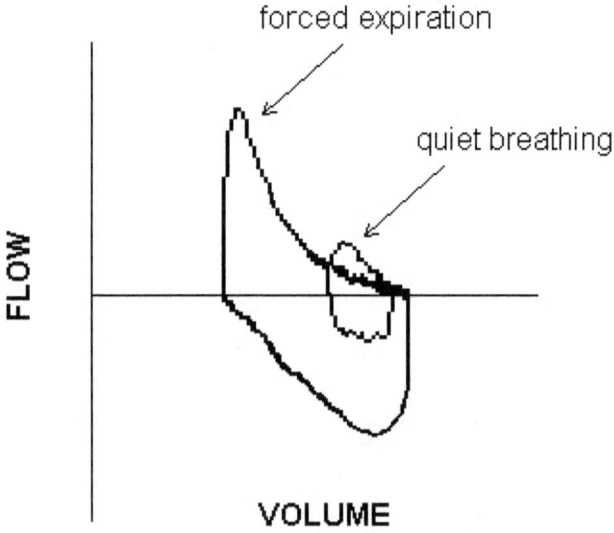

Figure 5-3. Flow-volume loops showing expiratory flows during quiet breathing that are higher than the expiratory flows during the forced expiration at the same lung volume.

In patients with a localized obstruction of the major airways, the typical shape of the F-V curve may change for plateaus either in the inspiratory or the expiratory limbs, or in both, depending on the characteristics of the obstruction (fixed or variable), and the location of the obstructing lesion (extrathoracic or intrathoracic).

When the obstruction in the major airways is fixed, i.e., does not change with the phases of respiration (e.g. neoplastic lesions), peak flows of both expiratory and inspiratory limbs are decreased in about equal proportions. The typical shape of the expiratory and inspiratory limbs is lost, and plateaus may be observed in both phases of respiration instead (Figure 5-4). This may happen if the lesions are either extrathoracic or intrathoracic.

If the obstruction is variable, i.e. it changes in magnitude according to the mechanics of breathing during inspiration and expiration (e.g. tracheomalacia), the pattern of the F-V loops is different in extrathoracic and intrathoracic lesions (Figure 5-4).

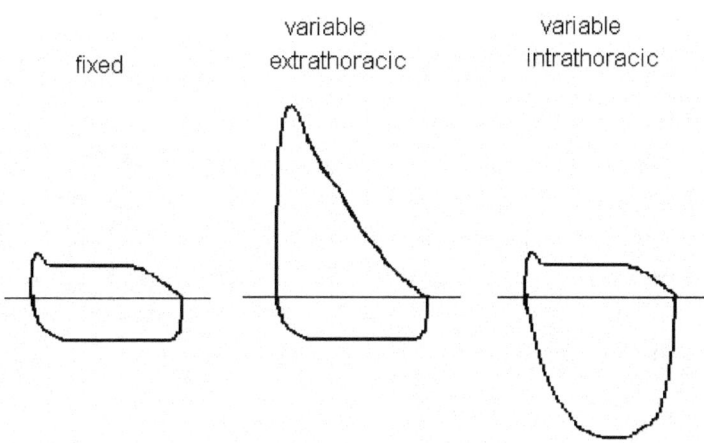

Figure 5-4. Characteristic F-V loops seen in patients with a localized obstruction of the major airways.

In variable extrathoracic lesions, there is a predominant distortion of the inspiratory loop, whereas in variable intrathoracic lesions there is a predominant distortion of the expiratory loop (Figure 5-4).

The effect of posture has been proposed as an additional factor to take into consideration when the shape of F-V curve is analyzed in the search of a pattern of variable airway obstruction of the major airways. The presence of any extrinsic mass near to the upper airways (e.g. thyroid goiter) may cause airway obstruction due to compression.[34] The degree of the airway compression may change with body posture. The F-V loops may fail to show evidence of upper airway flow limitation in the upright posture, and to demonstrate it in various recumbent positions. This could be particularly relevant to patients with respiratory symptoms when recumbent.[34]

Numeric results

Current computerized spirometers can provide a list of many parameters calculated from a test of forced expiration. The following question may arise: which variables should be considered for the interpretation?

Despite their interest in some physiological studies, the number of test parameters used in spirometry interpretation should be limited in the clinical area and epidemiological studies to avoid an excessive number of false positive results.[35] The parameters recommended by the American Thoracic Society and the European Respiratory Society [36] as the primary guides are:

1) Forced vital capacity (FVC).

2) Forced expiratory volume in 1 second (FEV_1).

3) Forced expiratory volume in 1 second to forced vital capacity ratio (FEV_1/FVC).

SPIROMETRY

There is a fourth parameter, the forced expiratory flow between the 25% and 75% of the FVC ($FEF_{25-75\%}$), which can be useful for the interpretation of borderline tests.

Chapter 6 is entirely dedicated to the analysis of the numeric results in spirometry tests.

Chapter 6

WHAT DO ALL THESE NUMBERS MEAN?

In the analysis of the numeric results, only the following parameters will be considered for spirometry interpretation: forced vital capacity (FVC), forced expiratory volume in 1 second (FEV_1), forced expiratory volume in 1 second to forced vital capacity ratio (FEV_1/FVC) and forced expiratory flow between 25% and 75% of the FVC ($FEF_{25-75\%}$). All other parameters that can be listed in a spirometry report are ignored here.

Reference (predicted) values

Values of the spirometry parameters measured in a test do not provide too much information unless we can determine whether the numbers are within normal limits. The values measured in an individual can be evaluated by comparison with the distribution of measurements in a reference healthy population of similar anthropometric characteristics (sex, age, height, and ethnic group). Logically, reference values should correspond to the anthropometric characteristics of the subject whose ventilatory function is being tested and, ideally, developed from normal subjects belonging to the same ethnic group.

Many reference equations have been published for different race/ethnic groups. Equations of linear regressions have been the most common way to describe the variations in pulmonary parameters with sex, age, height and race. However, the performance of such equations is less satisfactory at the edges of the data distribution. More complex equations have also been used to describe pulmonary function data, and the predicted values they provide are usually closer to those observed in the population from which the equations were derived. More recently, a new approach to modeling spirometry data, which produces "all age" reference curves has been introduced.[37] This approach allowed deriving continuous prediction equations to calculate predicted values for spirometry parameters as well as their lower limits of normal. These equations have been developed for different ethnic groups. In this work with use predicted values calculated with these multi-ethnic reference values for spirometry.[38]

A spirometry reference value calculator based on these equations can be found on-line at the following Internet address:

http://www.ers-education.org/guidelines/global-lung-function-initiative/tools.aspx

Lower limits of normal

The lower limits of normal are used to determine if the parameters measured in a particular patient are within normal limits. For a long time, the most common way of defining the normal values has been using a fixed percentage of measured values in relation to predicted (reference) values, e.g. to consider a measured value of a particular parameter at or above 80% of the predicted value as normal. This practice of using a fixed percentage value may work in children, but has no statistical basis in adults. In spirometry, measured values which are above the fifth percentile are considered to be within the normal or expected range.

Measured values falling below the fifth percentile are considered abnormal. However, lower limits of normal (LLN) should not be considered as absolute boundaries that correctly classify all patients into normal and abnormal groups. This is particularly true for subjects whose ventilatory function is close to the lower limits. LLN alone do not allow predicting the possibility of a lung disease. For these reasons, whenever it is possible, spirometry interpretation should be made using clinical information.

Spirometry patterns

To interpret a spirometry test, we first analyze each measured parameter, and then the final interpretation is made while considering all parameters as a group. In a composite made up of the different spirometry parameters considered in this analysis, the different possible combinations of normal and decreased (abnormal) values in a test are called the spirometry "patterns". Let us further explain this point using an analysis like the one shown in Table 6-1. We successively analyze the values of FVC, FEV_1/FVC, FEV_1 and $FEF_{25-75\%}$ measured in a test by comparing them with the lower limit of normal (LLN) for each parameter, according to the anthropometric characteristics of the subject, as explained in the previous section. In the case shown in Table 6-1, all the measured parameters are higher than their respective LLN. Hence, we arrive to the conclusion that the spirometry test is normal. However, the conclusion is not based on one parameter but on the analysis of all of them together. Table 6-1 represents the spirometry pattern of a normal test.

Indeed, the analysis of the results of any spirometry test can be made using the approach shown in Table 6-1. This is the approach used in this work to analyze the different spirometry patterns.

Table 6-1. Spirometry pattern of a normal test.

Parameter	Measured value is below the lower limit?	
	yes	no
FVC (L)		x
FEV1/FVC (%)		x
FEV1 (L)		x
FEV25-75% (L/s)		x
Interpretation	Normal spirometry test	

Let us show an example using numeric values. Table 6-2 shows the predicted values, lower limits of normal, and the measured values of the different parameters of a hypothetical spirometry test administered to a subject with the anthropometric characteristics described in the heading of the Table. The analysis made in Table 6-1 was added to Table 6-2. In this composite, all spirometry parameters are above the LLN. Therefore, we conclude that the test is normal.

The pattern of a normal spirometry test has been presented in this section. Spirometry patterns demonstrating abnormal spirometry tests are presented in the following sections.

Spirometry patterns with reduced FVC

As mentioned in Chapter 4, a restrictive ventilatory defect is characterized physiologically by a reduction in total lung capacity (TLC). The TLC cannot be measured by spirometry and, therefore, the FVC is used as a measure of lung replenishment. A restrictive defect is suspected when there is a reduced forced vital capacity and there is no evidence of airway obstruction. This is the spirometry 'restrictive' pattern. It should be noted that in this work the term restrictive **defect** will be used to designate the true abnormality within the respiratory system which could be detected by measuring the TLC, and the term restrictive **pattern** to indicate the spirogram with reduced FVC that may or may not reflect a true restrictive **defect** as will be explained below.

Table 6-2. Example of spirometry interpretation. Anthropometric data: sex, male; age, 45 yr; height, 175 cm; race/ethnic group, African-American.

Parameter	Predicted	Lower limit*	Measured	Measured value below the lower limit?	
				yes	no
FVC (L)	4.17	3.22	3.97		x
FEV1/FVC (%)	81	70	74		x
FEV1 (L)	3.36	2.56	2.93		x
FEF25-75% (L/s)	3.26	1.63	2.55		x
Interpretation	Normal spirometry test				

A spirometry test with a normal FVC practically excludes the diagnosis of a restrictive defect. However, when FVC is low, it cannot be assured that a restricitve defect is almost certainly present. It has been found that less than 60% of patients in a clinical population with the classical spirometric restrictive pattern have pulmonary restriction (restrictive defect) confirmed on lung volume measurements.[39] Therefore, a spirometry test with a restrictive pattern is only suggestive of the presence of a restrictive defect. If a spirometric restrictive pattern is observed in a patient with a disease expected to lead to small lung volumes, then the combination of spirometry plus clinical and other laboratory data will increase the accuracy of the diagnosis. In any case, it should be remembered that measurement of TLC is considered the "gold standard" for the diagnosis of a restrictive defect. In summary, if a spirometry test showing a restrictive pattern is the only pulmonary function test performed on a patient and there is clinical evidence of a disease leading to lung restriction, this should determine the necessity of further investigations, including lung volumes.

When FVC is low, a reduction of forced expiratory airflow measured by the absolute values of FEV_1 or $FEF_{25-75\%}$ could be simply the result of the small FVC. Thus, absolute values of FEV_1 or $FEF_{25-75\%}$ are not used as evidence of airway obstruction when FVC is decreased. For this reason, in this case, a measure of the maximal airflow from the lungs (usually measured by FEV_1) is compared to the maximal volume that can be displaced from the lungs (usually measured by FVC) to discover an airway obstruction, i.e., the FEV_1/FVC ratio. The presence of a reduced FVC along with a normal FEV_1/FVC ratio (i.e. no evidence of airway obstruction) is the classical restrictive spirometry pattern (Table 6-3).

Table 6-3. Restrictive spirometry pattern.

Parameter	Measured value is below the lower limit?	
	yes	no
FVC (L)	x	
FEV1/FVC (%)		x
FEV1 (L)	N/E*	
FEF25-75% (L/s)	N/E*	
Interpretation	Restrictive spirometry pattern suggesting a restrictive defect	

* N/E = Not evaluated. Low values could be simply the result of a small FVC.

A mixed ventilatory defect is present when abnormalities producing airway obstruction coexist with abnormalities leading to lung restriction in the same subject. However, the way this coexistence is reflected on a spirogram depends on the underlying abnormalities (see Chapter 4). It is not rare to observe spirograms with a combination of reduced FVC and evidence of airway obstruction. The limitations of FVC mentioned above for the detection of the pulmonary restriction are also present in this case. Keeping in mind the limitations of FVC and also the limitations of the absolute values of FEV_1 and $FEF_{25-75\%}$ for detecting airway obstruction in patients with reduced FVC, the mixed spirometry pattern is characterized by a reduced FVC coexisting with a reduced FEV_1/FVC ratio (Table 6-4).

Table 6-4. Mixed spirometry pattern.

Parameter	Measured value is below the lower limit?	
	yes	no
FVC (L)	x	
FEV1/FVC (%)	x	
FEV1 (L)	N/E*	
FEF25-75% (L/s)	N/E*	
Interpretation	Mixed spirometry pattern	

* N/E = Not evaluated. Low values could be simply the result of a small FVC.

When there is a mixed spirometry pattern, in many cases the decrease in FVC is not due to a true restrictive abnormality or defect but rather to gas trapping as a consequence of the airway obstruction. The gas trapping may produce an increase in the residual volume (RV) and a reduction in FVC while the total lung capacity (TLC) does not change significantly. The latter situation is often seen in asthmatic patients and also in patients with chronic obstructive pulmonary disease (COPD). Post-bronchodilator spirometry tests (see Chapter 7) may help to demonstrate the presence of gas trapping, if this is the case. Other tests of pulmonary function (lung volumes, and, in some subjects, respiratory mechanics) are recommended if they are justified by the clinic.

It should be remembered that the dynamic compression of the airways and expiratory flow limitation may be enhanced because of airway obstruction (see Chapter 3). In this situation, measurement of VC with slow maneuvers that both begin and end in nearly static efforts sometimes yields normal values of vital capacity when the measured FVC was below the lower limit of normal. In that case, the spirometry pattern with reduced FVC is no longer considered.

Obstructive spirometry patterns

An airway obstruction produces a decrease of maximal airflow from the lungs. As mentioned above, an obstructive ventilatory defect is better defined as a disproportionate reduction of the maximal airflow with respect to the maximal lung volume. For this reason, a decreased FEV_1/FVC is recommended as the primary guide for identifying an obstructive pattern. However, the interpretation of the presence of an obstructive abnormality in a spirometry test should be made also taking into consideration other parameters. In other words, there is not only one spirometry pattern that can be interpreted as showing an obstructive abnormality.

A classical obstructive spirometry pattern is the one characterized by normal FVC, decreased FEV_1, and low FEV_1/FVC (Table 6-5). When FEV_1/FVC is decreased, there is no need to evaluate the $FEF_{25-75\%}$, which most probably will be also decreased. The FEF_{25-}

75% is not evaluated in this case because it is a parameter with more intra-individual variability than FEV_1/FVC. When FEV_1/FVC is decreased, if a normal value of $FEF_{25-75\%}$ coexisted it is disregarded.

Table 6-5. Obstructive spirometry pattern.

Parameter	Measured value is below the lower limit?	
	yes	no
FVC (L)		x
FEV1/FVC (%)	x	
FEV1 (L)	x	
FEF25-75% (L/s)	N/E*	
Interpretation	Obstructive abnormality	

* N/E = Not evaluated. When FEV1/FVC is decreased, there is no need to evaluate the FEF25-75%.

The FEV_1/FVC is the primary guide for identifying an obstructive pattern, but there are exceptions to this general rule. A FEV_1/FVC ratio below the lower limit of normal along with a value of FEV_1 within the normal range can be observed, and this pattern does not necessarily means that there is a pulmonary impairment. Indeed, a low FEV_1/FVC ratio along with FEV_1 values which are equal to or above predicted can be seen in healthy subjects such as athletes and workers in some physically demanding occupations.[35,40] This particular pattern has been considered a physiological variant. However, recent evidences demonstrate that to distinguish between a physiological variant and a mild obstructive abnormality, clinical information should be evaluated and other tests of respiratory function should be performed.[41,42] A pattern like the one shown in Table 6-6 should lead to a more detailed evaluation of the subject.

The presence of respiratory symptoms, bronchodilator reversibility or challenge test, and lung volume measurement may help to assist in detecting an early obstructive abnormality, or alternatively, to arrive to the conclusion that it is a physiological variant. A respiratory evaluation beyond spirometry should not be limited to those subjects with an FEV_1 above 100% of predicted value because the same pattern but with an FEV_1 below 100% of predicted value could also represent a normal physiological variant.[42] This distinction is of practical relevance because the treatment of obstructive pulmonary diseases is based on proper recognition of airflow obstruction.[41]

Table 6-6. Low FEV1/FVC and normal FEV1.

Parameter	Measured value is below the lower limit?	
	yes	no
FVC (L)		x
FEV1/FVC (%)	x	
FEV1 (L)		x
FEF25-75% (L/s)	N/E*	
Interpretation	Mild obstructive abnormality or a physiological variant. More tests.	

* N/E = Not evaluated. When FEV1/FVC is decreased, there is no need to evaluate the FEF25-75%.

There is another exception to the general rule of using the FEV_1/FVC ratio to interpret the presence of an airway obstruction. There is a situation in which FEV_1/FVC is normal but very close to or at the lower limit or normal. In this case, the $FEF_{25\text{-}75\%}$ may help to determine whether the test can be interpreted as showing the presence of an airway obstruction. Early changes associated with airflow obstruction in the airways are better reflected in the terminal portion of the volume-time spirogram (which is evaluated by the measurement of FEF25-75%) even when the initial part of the volume-time spirogram (where FEV1 is measured) is barely affected. Test results with FVC, FEV1, and FEV1/FVC within normal limits but borderline FEV1/FVC and low FEF25-75% suggest the presence of airway obstruction (Table 6-7).

The spirometry pattern presented in Table 6-7 can also be observed with a variant in which not only the FEF25-75% is decreased but also the FEV1. This spirometry pattern also suggests the presence of airway obstruction (Table 6-8).

Table 6-7. Obstructive spirometry pattern.

Parameter	Measured value is below the lower limit?	
	yes	no
FVC (L)		x
FEV1/FVC (%)		x
FEV1 (L)		x
FEF25-75% (L/s)	x	
Interpretation	Obstructive abnormality	

This section about obstructive spirometry patterns is an appropriate place to mention another situation illustrating the importance of clinical information in spirometry interpretation. There are subjects, such as asthmatic patients, in whom we expect to find an obstructive spirometry pattern. However, it is possible to observe in these patients the spirometry pattern of reduced FVC with normal FEV_1/FVC which is the characteristic restrictive spirometry pattern (Table 6-3). A possible explanation to this is that there has been a patchy collapse of small airways early in the expiration which has produced gas trapping, increased residual volume, and reduced FVC. Knowledge of the obstructive antecedents in the subject will make us think on this possibility and try to demonstrate its presence. In these cases, measurement of the slow vital capacity (VC) may give a more correct estimation of the vital capacity and hence of the obstructive impairment, which should be evaluated in this case by the FEV_1/VC ratio and not the FEV_1/FVC ratio. Also, a post-bronchodilator test may help to put in evidence the obstruction. In some asthmatic subjects, the low FVC may even increase to values within the normal limits after a bronchodilator, hence excluding a restrictive defect.[43]

Table 6-8. Obstructive spirometry pattern.

Parameter	Measured value is below the lower limit?	
	yes	no
FVC (L)		x
FEV1/FVC (%)		x
FEV1 (L)	x	
FEF25-75% (L/s)	x	
Interpretation	Obstructive abnormality	

Isolated FEV₁ reduction

Lastly, there is a spirometry pattern that is rarely reported but possible to observe. This is the case of an isolated decrease in FEV₁. This spirometry pattern requires, in first instance, to repeat the test (Table 6-9). The spirometry pattern of an isolated decrease in FEV₁ could result from an expiratory maneuver that ended prematurely in a subject with an obstructive impairment. In this situation, FVC is underestimated and the FEV1/FVC relationship is artificially increased and falls in the normal range. Also as a consequence of the expiratory maneuver that ended prematurely, FEF$_{25-75\%}$ is measured at a higher lung volume, yielding a normal value.

However, this unusual spirometry pattern may still be observed when the test has been performed correctly. The pattern may occur in a situation in which the FVC of the subject is within the normal range but very close to the lower limit of normal, probably due to the progressive installation of a restrictive defect that has not decreased FVC sufficiently to make it fall into the abnormal range. This spirometry pattern illustrates the point that lower limits of normal should not be considered as absolute boundaries that correctly classify all patients into normal and abnormal groups, particularly when parameters' values are close to lower limits.

Table 6-9. Isolated FEV1 reduction.

Parameter	Measured value is below the lower limit?	
	yes	no
FVC (L)		x
FEV1/FVC (%)		x
FEV1 (L)	x	
FEF25-75% (L/s)		x
Interpretation	Unusual pattern. More tests	

A recent study analyzing retrospectively clinical, spirometry and radiological data from 15,192 subjects who underwent a medical check-up, found that 323 (2.1%) had an isolated FEV1 reduction (the authors analyzed FVC, FEV1, and FEV1/FVC data).[44] Compared with the group of subjects with normal spirometry (69.7%), those with isolated FEV1 reduction had more frequently a history of respiratory disease (8.4% vs. 3.0%) and more radiological abnormalities (15.5% vs. 4.3%). The radiological abnormalities most frequently found were pleural thickening and inactive tuberculosis.[44]

It should be kept in mind that, whenever it is possible, spirometry interpretation should be made using clinical information or other data to best support clinical decision making. In the case of an isolated decrease in FEV1, other respiratory tests should be performed.

Severity classification of ventilatory impairments in spirometry

So far, we have seen spirometry patterns showing ventilatory impairments. However, an evaluation about the severity of the abnormality has not been mentioned. The degree of severity of a ventilatory impairment is, in general, associated with patients' respiratory complaints, morbidity and prognosis. However, the symptoms or prognosis of individual patients cannot be accurately predicted from spirometry parameters. Nevertheless, an important element in spirometry interpretation is to provide a severity classification for an abnormality observed in the test results.

For obstructive impairments, we have seen above that absolute values of FEV1 are not usually used **to detect** airway obstruction, and that the FEV1/FVC is the primary parameter that should be used. However, **for classifying** the severity of an obstructive impairment, we should use the FEV1 and not the FEV1/FVC ratio. The reason for that is that both FEV1 and FVC may decrease with the progression of disease. This way, for example, an FEV1/FVC ratio of 60% may correspond to FEV1 of

1.8 L with FVC of 3.0 L, but also to FEV_1 of 1.2 L with FVC of 2 L; in the same subject, the second situation indicates more impairment than the first one. For this reason, the classification of an obstructive lung function impairment should be based on the FEV_1 expressed in percent of the predicted value (FEV_1 % pred = [measured FEV_1/predicted FEV_1] x 100).

Not only in obstructive impairments, but also in both restrictive and mixed abnormalities severity classification of lung function impairment should be based on the FEV_1 expressed in percent of the predicted value. The justification for this is that when there is a reduction in FVC due to a restrictive abnormality, the FEV_1 is also necessarily reduced, but if there is a concomitant obstructive abnormality, the FEV_1 is reduced even more.

Due to the reasons explained above, the ATS and the ERS recommend the use of the FEV_1 expressed in percent of the predicted value (FEV_1 % pred) to estimate the severity of any spirometric abnormality.[36] Table 6-10 shows a proposed severity classification where the cut-off points are arbitrary. Other categorizations with different cut-off points may also be used.

Use of the general rule shown in Table 6-10 to classify the severity of an airway obstruction has an exception. As explained in Chapter 5, there are two main types of airway obstruction: diffused airway obstruction in the bronchial tree and upper airway obstruction (UAO). In the patients with UOA, the severity classification used in Table 6-10 may have little applicability because patients may have life-threatening conditions (e.g. a tracheal stenosis) which do not produce a marked decrease in FEV_1 and spirometry test results might even be classified as mild obstruction, not reflecting the severity of the situation. In these cases, the shape of the flow-volume curve (see Chapter 5) and clinical data will allow a correct interpretation of spirometry results.

Table 6-10. Severity classification of any ventilatory abnormality (obstructive, restrictive or mixed) detected by spirometry.

Range of FEV1 % pred	Severity
$\geq$ 70 %	Mild
60 % - 69 %	Moderate
50 % - 59 %	Moderately severe
49 % - 35 %	Severe
< 35 %	Very severe

Chapter 7

BRONCHODILATOR RESPONSE

Airway responsiveness to a bronchodilator is often tested to assist in the diagnosis of asthma and to assess the amount of reversibility present in cases of chronic airflow limitation.

FEV_1 and FVC should be the primary guides to judge bronchodilator response. However, there is controversy on what constitutes reversibility in subjects with airway obstruction, and on how a bronchodilator response should be expressed. Three common methods of expressing a bronchodilator response are:

1. Absolute change (in liters or ml) in FEV_1 and/or FVC.
2. Percent of the initial (baseline) FEV_1 and/or FVC value calculated as (post-value - pre-value)/pre-value.
3. Percent of the predicted value calculated as (post-value - pre-value)/predicted value.

The ATS and ERS recommend considering an improvement in an individual subject only if the percent change **and** absolute change in FEV_1 or FVC are clearly beyond the expected variability of the measurement during a single test session. It is required at least a 12 % increase in FEV_1 or FVC from the baseline values, and an absolute change of 200 ml (as long as the increase in FVC is not the result of a longer expiratory time) to define a meaningful response (Figure 7-1).[36]

It has been reported that expressing the change in FEV1 or FVC as percent of the predicted value has advantages over the percent of the initial value.[45] The predicted values after inhalation of a bronchodilator may be less subject to bias than measuring percent change from baseline and may have a higher likelihood of separating patients who have asthma from those who have COPD. In this case, an increase in FEV1 or FVC greater than 6% can be considered significant.[46]

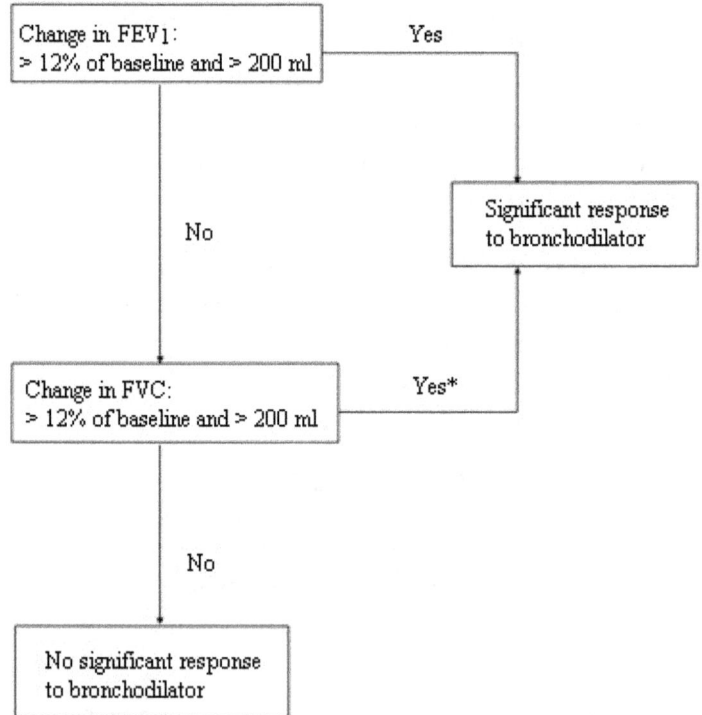

*Caution: changes in FVC must not be due to a longer expiratory time.

Figure 7-1. Algorithm for interpreting a response to bronchodilator.

The $FEF_{25-75\%}$ should be considered only as a secondary option to evaluate a bronchodilator response. If used, it must be taken into account that after inhalation of a bronchodilator aerosol or any other bronchodilator treatment, changes in FVC and TLC can modify the volume at which the pre- and post-treatment values of $FEF_{25-75\%}$ are measured. If FVC changes after the administration of a bronchodilator, then any variation between pre- and post-treatment values of $FEF_{25-75\%}$ cannot be attributed solely to a change in airway obstruction. A decrease of $FEF_{25-75\%}$ when other indices of obstruction improve can be observed after a bronchodilator treatment. This paradoxical worsening is an artifact in the calculation. It most often occurs because after treatment the $FEF_{25-75\%}$ is measured at lower absolute lung volumes, where there is less elastic distension of the intrathoracic airways. This can happen because of the presence of either one or both of the following mechanisms:

1) The bronchodilator therapy may increase the forced vital capacity because of the decreased residual volume, and this lowers the absolute lung volumes covered by the middle part of the FVC curve where $FEF_{25-75\%}$ is measured (Figure 7-2).
2) With the bronchodilator response the TLC may decrease because of the opening of airways and the release of some volume of gas previously trapped, causing all measurements from the FVC curve to be taken at lower absolute lung volumes.

It has been proposed to measure what is called isovolume $FEF_{25-75\%}$ to compare pre- and post-treatment values of $FEF_{25-75\%}$ when FVC increases after use of a bronchodilator.[47] The method consists in marking points on the post-treatment FVC curves at identical volumes down from the starting point of the curve as on the pre-treatment FVC curve (Figure 7-2). The slope of the line connecting these points, isovolume $FEF_{25-75\%}$, is the parameter used for comparison. It has been claimed that measurement of isovolume $FEF_{25-75\%}$ whenever FVC increases acutely after use of a bronchodilator improves recognition of responses otherwise missed.[47]

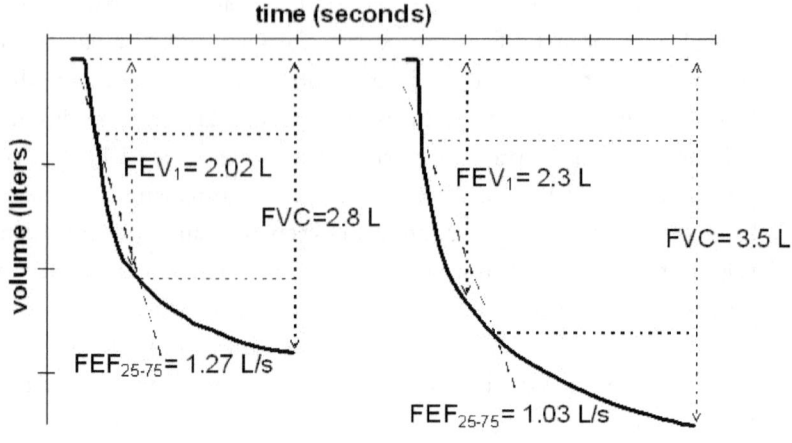

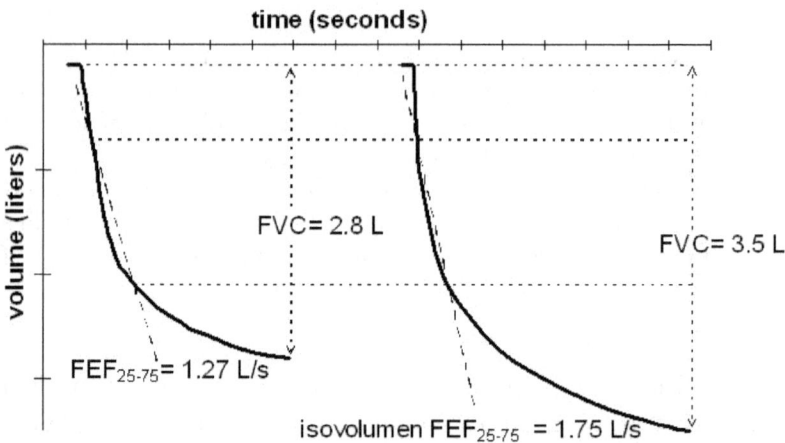

Figure 7-2. Comparison of pre- (left) and post-treatment (right) values of FEF25-75% when the vital capacity increases after use of a bronchodilator. *Top*: measurement of FEF25-75% without taking into account the change in lung volume. *Bottom*: measurement of the isovolume FEF25-75%.

Persistent airway obstruction after a bronchodilator test

It is important to underline that a patient who did not have a significant bronchodilator response in a single laboratory testing session may respond to long-term bronchodilator therapy. Therefore, a single test of bronchodilator response is not adequate to assess neither the underlying airway responsiveness nor the potential for therapeutic benefits of bronchodilator therapy. Repeating the spirometry test after a long-term therapy with bronchodilators and/or steroids may provide better information about the reversibility of the obstructive impairment.

The hallmark of bronchial asthma is airway obstruction reversibility. However, long-tem, unresolved airway inflammation in asthma can result in permanent structural changes in the airways called 'remodeling'. Structural changes in remodeling include increased airway wall thickness that involves smooth muscle and collagen tissue, increased mucous glands and mucus production and increased blood vessels in the airways. Remodeling may produce variable degrees of irreversible obstruction in asthmatic patients with long evolution.

Chronic obstructive lung disease (COPD) is characterized by a limitation to airflow that is not fully reversible. The airway obstruction in COPD is associated with remodeling and inflammatory cellular infiltrate in small airways, destruction of alveoli and enlargement of airspaces. Patients with COPD can be classified according to the Global Initiative for Chronic Obstructive Lung Disease (GOLD) classification that is based on the results of post-bronchodilator spirometry tests.[48] However, it should be noted that the GOLD classification is based on fixed percentages of FEV_1 and FEV_1/FVC. Normal or predicted values of these parameters decrease with age in adult subjects. Therefore, use of fixed values to establish the presence of irreversible airway obstruction may underestimate the presence of obstruction in young adults and overestimate airway obstruction in the elderly.

Chapter 8

INTERRELATIONSHIP OF SPIROMETRY PARAMETERS: A GRAPHICAL APPROACH

Spirometry parameters may change in different ways, depending on the pathologic conditions that cause the ventilatory changes. The different variations of the parameters result in various spirometry patterns (see Chapter 6). Although spirometry parameters may change differently, interrelationship among them exists. Probably, the best-known example of this interrelationship is that when FVC increases or decreases, similar changes usually occur in FEV_1 too. In this chapter, a graphic representation of the simultaneous variations of the basic spirometry parameters is developed to allow a visual analysis of the interrelationship among them. A reader that is not interested in following the development of the graph may go directly to Figures 8-2, 8-3 and 8-7 and analyze the situations shown in Figures 8-4, 8-5, 8-8, 8-9, and 8-10.

Analysis and interpretation of the forced expiratory spirogram should be based, at least, on 3 basic parameters: FVC, FEV_1 and the FEV_1/FVC ratio. The $FEF_{25-75\%}$ will be considered here as the fourth parameter. Another parameter, the $FEF_{25-75\%}/FVC$ ratio, is also used in the development of the graphic representation of the simultaneous variations of the parameters. The $FEF_{25-75\%}/FVC$ ratio has the units of reciprocal time (seg^{-1}).

The FEF$_{25\text{-}75\%}$/FVC ratio has been used as a surrogate measure of airway size relative to lung size (which is called dysanapsis) because FEF$_{25\text{-}75\%}$ is sensitive to airway size, and FVC is sensitive to lung size.[49] But essentially, the FEF$_{25\text{-}75\%}$/FVC ratio is an expression of the speed (in the middle half of FVC) with which the lung is emptying. Both FEV$_1$/FVC and FEF$_{25\text{-}75\%}$/FVC ratios are expressions of lung emptying; therefore, it is not surprising to find that there is a relationship between them.

Using spirometry data from different groups of subjects, the graphic representation of the relationship between FEF$_{25\text{-}75\%}$/FVC and FEV$_1$/FVC yields a non-linear distribution similar to the one shown in Figure 8-1. A FEF$_{25\text{-}75\%}$/FVC vs. FEV$_1$/FVC relationship like the one shown in Figure 8-1 can be obtained using data from subjects of different age, sex, height, ethnic group and ventilatory function in the same sample. However, it is necessary to use a sample of subjects with a range of ventilatory function that goes from normal to very low lung function to be able to observe a non-linear distribution of points in the relationship. When FEF$_{25\text{-}75\%}$/FVC is placed in the ordinate (x axis) and FEV$_1$/FVC in the abscissa (y axis), the relationship is best fitted by an exponential function with the general form:

$$\text{FEF}_{25\text{-}75\%}/\text{FVC} = a\, e^{b\, \text{FEV}_1/\text{FVC}} \qquad \text{equation 1}$$

In equation 1, a and b are the coefficients of the equation, and e is a constant equal to 2.718281. For the exponential regression curve that was calculated with the sample of subjects shown in Figure 8-1, the coefficients a and b were 0.02 and 4.506, respectively, and the correlation coefficient (r) was 0.974. Therefore, the regression equation of the exponential curve shown in Figure 8-1 is as follows:

$$\text{FEF}_{25\text{-}75\%}/\text{FVC} = 0.02\, (2.718281)^{4.506\, \text{FEV}_1/\text{FVC}} \qquad \text{equation 2}$$

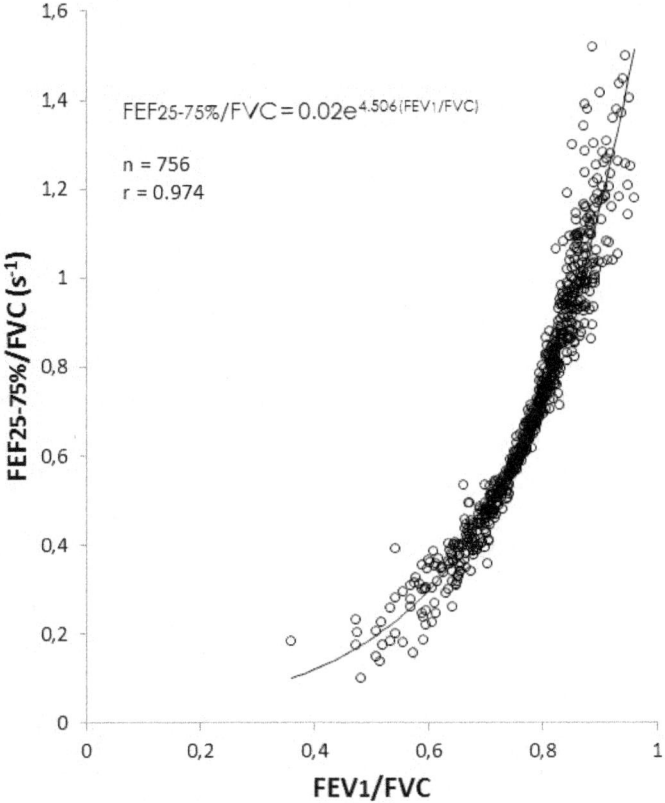

Figure 8-1. FEF25-75%/FVC vs. FEV1/FVC relationship obtained in a group of subjects with different age, sex, race and ventilatory function. The curve represents the exponential regression curve fitting best the data.

One obtains the same exponential distribution and a similar calculated exponential regression equation, with little variation of coefficients *a* and *b* and always with a high correlation coefficient (r), when using different samples of subjects,. It should be remembered that that there must be a wide range of ventilatory function in the subjects of the sample to be able to observe the non-linear distribution of points in the relationship.

Solving equation 2 for $FEF_{25-75\%}$, we are left with the following expression:

$$FEF_{25-75\%} = FVC\ [0.02\ (2.718281)^{4.506\ FEV_1/FVC}] \quad \text{equation 3}$$

Equation 3 allows us to estimate approximately the $FEF_{25-75\%}$ from a spirometry test whenever FEV_1 and FVC are known. It should be noted that the $FEF_{25-75\%}$ estimated with equation 3 may differ somehow from the actual $FEF_{25-75\%}$ measured in the same spirometry test from which FVC and FEV_1 were taken. This is because the regression equation used for the estimation is not a perfect representation of all the actual values used in its calculation. However, usually there is not a big difference between measured and estimated values of $FEF_{25-75\%}$ and, therefore, the estimated value is good enough for an analysis of the interaction of $FEF_{25-75\%}$ with FVC, FEV_1 and FEV_1/FVC.

In equation 3, $FEF_{25-75\%}$ is expressed as a function of FEV_1/FVC and FVC. However, the equation can also be used to estimate changes in FEV_1 and $FEF_{25-75\%}$ when there is a ventilatory abnormality that does not affect FVC, i.e. to obtain $FEF_{25-75\%}$ vs. FEV_1 relationships at any particular value of FVC. We can do it calculating $FEF_{25-75\%}$ at different values of FEV_1 while leaving FVC constant. For example, the equation describing the relationship between $FEF_{25-75\%}$ and FEV_1 when FVC is 4 L would be the following:

$$FEF_{25-75\%} = 4\ [0.02\ (2.718281)^{4.506\ FEV_1/4}]$$
equation 4

We can construct a graphic representation of the $FEF_{25-75\%}$ vs. FEV_1 relationship when FVC is 4 L by using different values of FEV_1 in equation 4 and calculating the corresponding values of $FEF_{25-75\%}$. Such graphic representation is shown in Figure 8-2.

SPIROMETRY

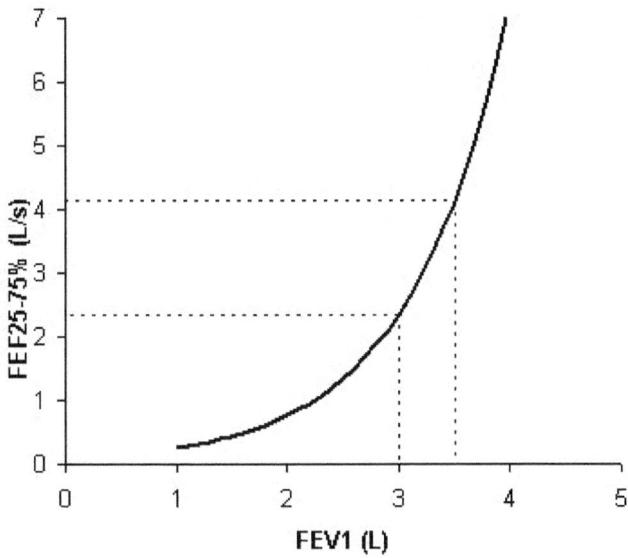

Figure 8-2. Interrelationship of parameters. When FVC remains constant, any increase or decrease in FEV1 is accompanied by an increase or decrease of FEF25-75% in a way that follows an exponential curve. In the upper part of the curve, any change in FEV1 is associated to a bigger change in FEF25-75%.

It is possible to repeat the same procedure described keeping FVC constant but using different values of FVC, and construct a graph showing a group of iso-FVC curves (curves representing constant FVC) or FVC isopleths in the $FEF_{25-75\%}$ vs. FEV_1 relationship. Figure 8-3 shows FVC isopleths for FVC values from 1.5 L to 6.5 L at intervals of FVC of 0.5 L. Each curve was drawn estimating the $FEF_{25-75\%}$ values for a range of FEV_1 from $FEV_1 = 0.3$ up to $FEV_1 = FVC$. Exceptions to this upper limit are isopleths for FVC values of 4 L or bigger, where the maximal value of FEV1 used was the one yielding an estimated $FEF_{25-75\%} = 7$ L/s, that was arbitrarily set as the upper limit for the y axis.

As mentioned before, the interrelationship among FVC, FEV1

and FEF25-75% shown in Figure 8-3 is an approximation due to the fact that the equation 3 used to construct the graph only approximates the distribution of points in the FEF25-75%/FVC vs. FEV1/FVC relationship. However, due to the high correlation coefficient between the variables, the figure provides a good approximation of their interrelationship and allows a better understanding of some changes observed in spirometry tests, as shown in Figures 8-4 and 8-5.

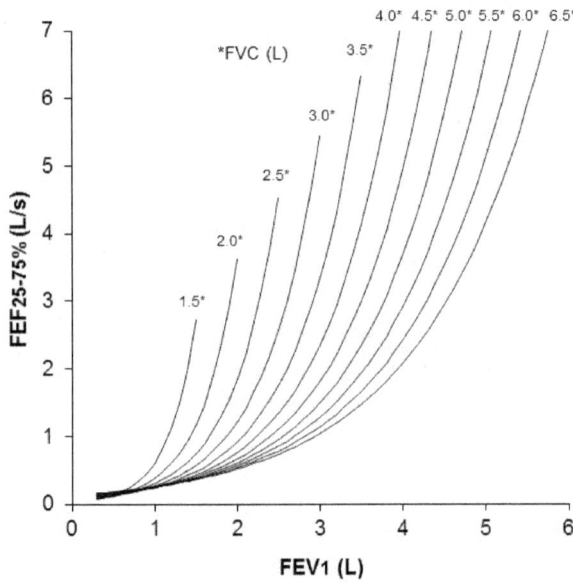

Figure 8-3. Group of FVC isopleths (constant FVC in each curve) in the FEF25-75% vs. FEV1 relationship.

However, Figure 8-3 lacks the information regarding FEV1/FVC which is a key parameter in spirometry testing. To include FEV1/FVC in figure 8-3, it is necessary to identify in each FVC isopleth the points corresponding to the same FEV1/FVC ratio, i.e. isoFEV1/FVC points. Such points differ from one FVC isopleth to the other. Some examples of how isoFEV1/FVC points can be identified are shown in table 8-1.

SPIROMETRY

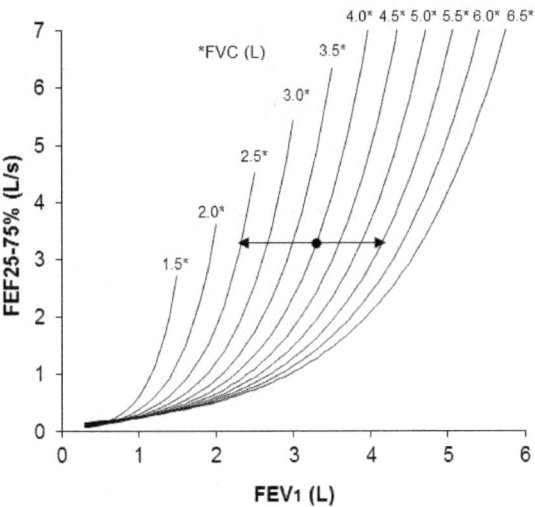

Figure 8-4. Interrelationship of parameters. Arrows in the figure show that a decrease or an increase in FEV1 may occur without any change in FEF25-75%, as long as FVC decreases or increases too.

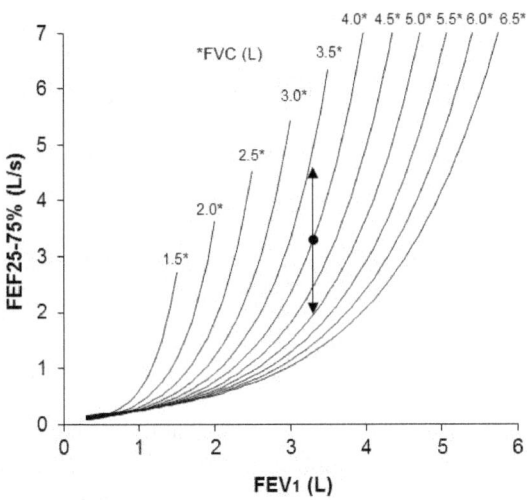

Figure 8-5. Interrelationship of parameters. FEF25-75% may decrease and FEV1 remain constant if there were a simultaneous increase in FVC, and vice versa.

Table 8-1. Example of calculation of isoFEV1/FVC points for different FVC isopleths in the FEF25-75% vs. FEV1 relationship.

FVC (L)	FEV1/FVC (%)	FEV1 (L)	FEF25-75%* (L/s)
1.5	90	90% of 1.5 = 1.35	1.73
2.0	90	90% of 2.0 =1.80	2.31
2.5	90	90% of 2.5 =2.25	2.89
3.0	90	90% of 3.0 = 2.70	3.46
1.5	80	80% of 1.5 = 1.20	1.10
2.0	80	80% of 2.0 =1.60	1.47
2.5	80	80% of 2.5 =2.00	1.84
3.0	80	80% of 3.0 = 2.40	2.21
1.5	70	70% of 1.5 = 1.05	0.70
2.0	70	70% of 2.0 = 1.40	0.94
2.5	70	70% of 2.5 = 1.75	1.17
3.0	70	70% of 3.0 = 2.10	1.41

*Calculated using Equation 3.

The isoFEV$_1$/FVC points are indeed FEV$_1$ values within each FVC. For example, if we are interested in FEV$_1$/FVC = 70%, the isoFEV$_1$/FVC point when FVC is 2.0 L is calculated as 70% of 2.0, that is, the value of FEV$_1$ when it is 70% of FVC (1.4 L in this case). Then we calculate FEF$_{25-75\%}$ using Equation 3 to bring this value to the graph FEF$_{25-75\%}$ vs. FEV$_1$.

Figure 8-6 shows the isoFEV1/FVC points for FEV1/FVC = 70% in different FVC isopleths. Once the isoFEV1/FVC points have been identified on each FVC isopleth, it is possible to join them to obtain isoFEV1/FVC lines or FEV1/FVC isopleths.

The result of doing such procedure for several values of FEV1/FVC is shown in Figure 8-7. The graph in Figure 8-7, which can be called the FEF25-75%-FEV1 diagram, represents a tool to visually analyze the interrelationships among the main spirometry parameters. The graph may be helpful for teaching and may provide guidance for interpreting different spirometry patterns. The analysis of different situations of the interaction of FVC, FEV1, FEV1/FVC and FEF25-75% can be observed in Figures 8-8, 8-9 and 8-10.

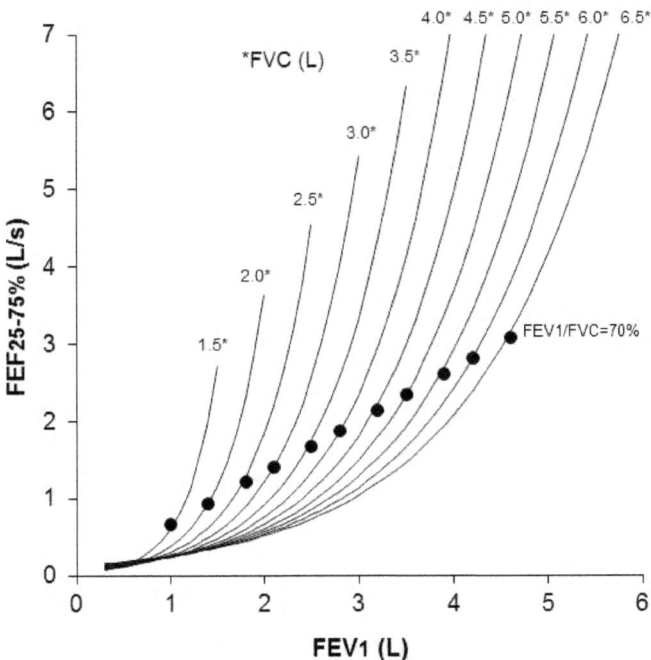

Figure 8-6. FEF25-75% vs. FEV1 relationship showing a group of FVC isopleths and the points corresponding to FEV1/FVC = 70% on each isopleth.

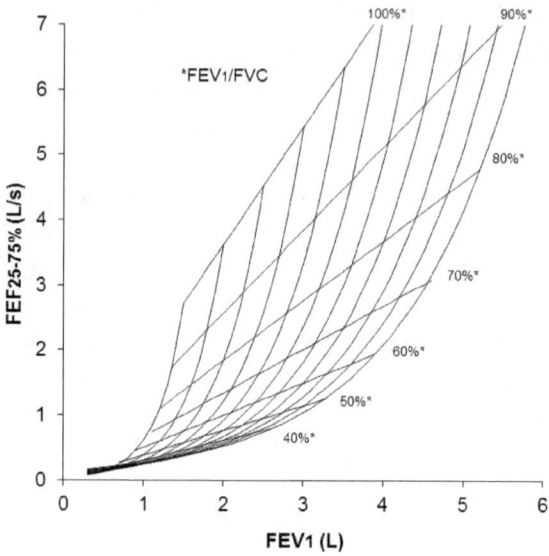

Figure 8-7. The FEF25-75%-FEV1 diagram showing a group of FVC isopleths (exponential curves) and FEV1/FVC isopleths (straight lines).

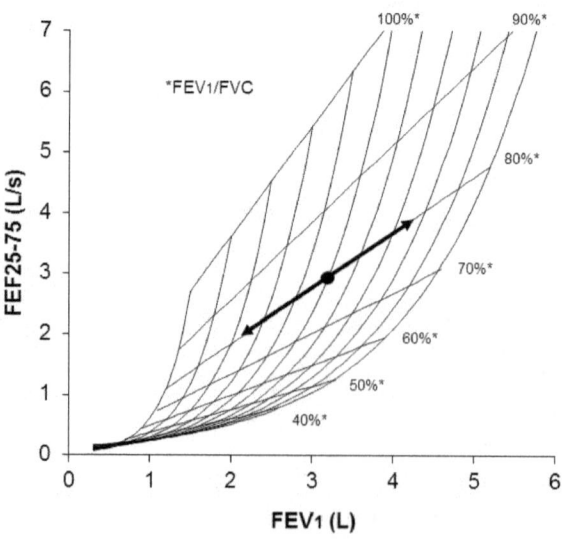

Figure 8-8. Interrelationship of parameters. Arrows were included in the figure to illustrate changes that may occur in the spirometry pattern when FEV1/FVC remains constant.

SPIROMETRY

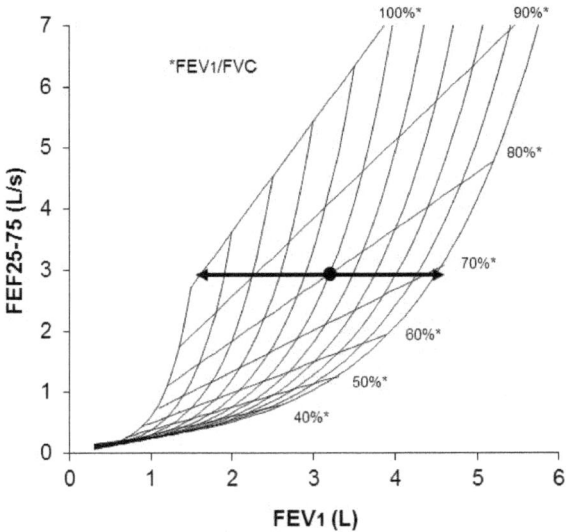

Figure 8-9. Interrelationship of parameters. The arrows illustrate that the FEV1/FVC ratio may increase and FEF25-75% may remain constant while both FVC and FEV1 decrease. Also, the FEV1/FVC ratio may decrease and FEF25-75% may remain constant while both FVC and FEV1 increase.

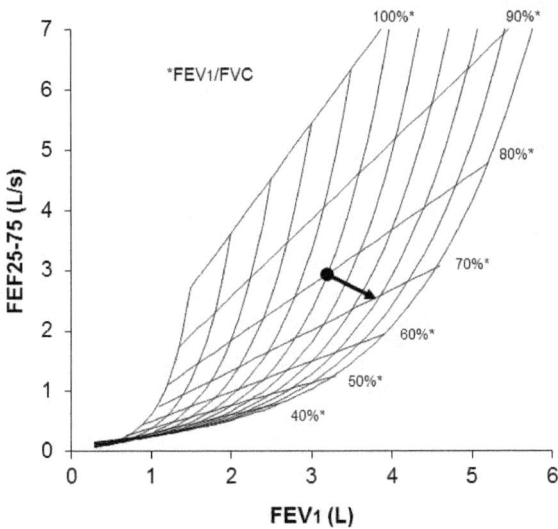

Figure 8-10. Interrelationship of parameters. Both FVC and FEV1 may increase at the same time that FEF25-75% and FEV1/FVC decrease.

Chapter 9

INTERRELATIONSHIP OF SPIROMETRY PARAMETERS: GLOBAL LUNG FUNCTION 2012 REFERENCE VALUES

The derivation of continuous multi-ethnic equations from age 3 to 95 years for spirometry reference values,[38] provides an opportunity to test the generalizability of the interrelationship of spirometry parameters. The equations have made possible to calculate continuous predicted values of high quality while changing the variables age, sex, height, and ethnic group in different ways.

Predicted values of FVC, FEV$_1$, FVC/FEV$_1$ and FEF$_{25-75\%}$ were calculated for Caucasians, African-Americans, North-Eastern Asians, and South-Eastern Asians using the equations and tools provided by the Global Lung Function Initiative (http://www.ers-education.org/guidelines/global-lung-function-initiative/tools.aspx).

Within each ethnic group, predicted values were calculated for male and female subjects from age 8 to 15 years at one year interval, and from 20 to 80 years at 10 years intervals. The values of height used in all ethnic groups were the same. For children from age 8 to 15 years, the values of height (in centimeters) used were:

Age (yrs.)	8	9	10	11	12	13	14	15
Height (cm.)	126	133	138	143	149	157	163	169

For adult male subjects from age 20 to 80, the height used was 175 cm; for adult female subjects in the same age interval, the height used was 162 cm. This way, 120 sets of predicted values were obtained. These sets can be considered either predicted values for a cross-sectional study with 120 subjects or predicted values for a longitudinal study with 8 subjects (one male and one female in each ethnic group) from age 8 to 80. As expected, predicted values of the different parameters of lung function varied among the 120 sets. Predicted values of FVC and $FEF_{25-75\%}$ were used to calculate the $FEF_{25-75\%}/FVC$ ratio for each subject. These calculated data were used to obtain a graphic of the $FEF_{25-75\%}/FVC$ vs. FEV_1/FVC relationship, and the distribution of points in the graph was compared with the exponential regression curve obtained in Figure 8-1, in the previous chapter. The result is shown in Figure 9-1.

It can be observed from Figure 9-1 that all predicted values fall on the steepest, upper part of the exponential curve that was obtained with another sample of subjects with a larger variation of lung function. Also, it can be observed that predicted values seem to follow a straight line. Therefore, a linear regression equation fitting the points was calculated. The calculated regression equation that best fitted all the points was:

$FEF_{25-75\%}/FVC = 4.056\ FEV_1/FVC - 2.515$ equation 1

The regression line drawn with equation 1 is shown in Figure 9-2.

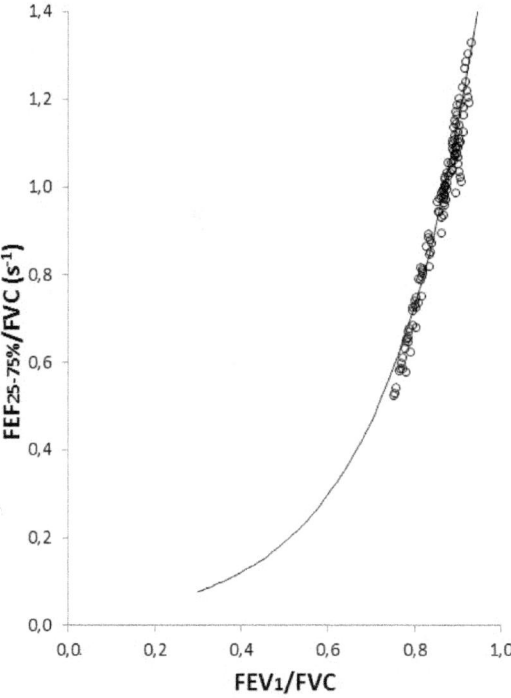

Figure 9-1. FEF25-75%/FVC vs. FEV1/FVC relationship obtained with the predicted values of four different ethnic groups in subjects with different age, sex and ventilatory function (see text for explanation). The curve represents the exponential regression curve obtained with a different sample that is shown in Figure 8-1 of the previous chapter.

Solving equation 1 for $FEF_{25-75\%}$, we are left with the following expression:

$FEF_{25-75\%}$ = FVC (4.056 FEV1/FVC − 2.515)   equation 2

Similar procedures to those used for the exponential regression equation in the proceeding chapter were applied to equation 2. This way, it was possible to construct a graph showing a group of iso-FVC lines (constant FVC in each particular line) or FVC isopleths in the $FEF_{25-75\%}$ vs. FEV1 relationship for predicted values (Figure 9-3).

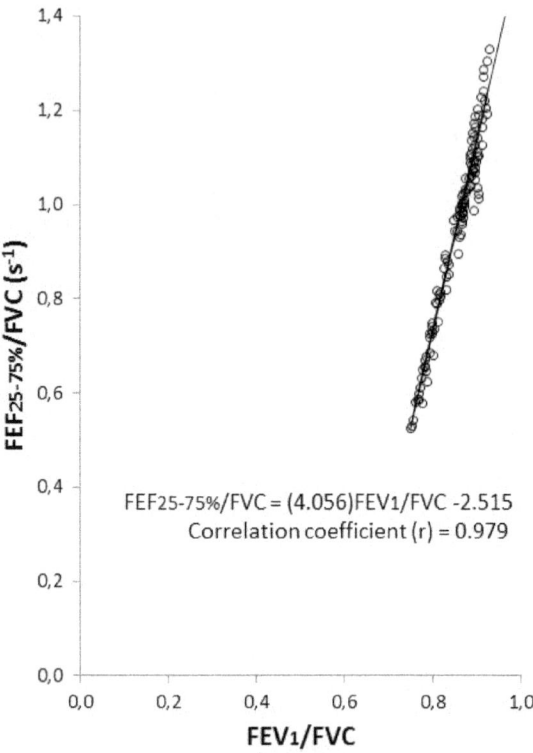

Figure 9-2. FEF25-75%/FVC vs. FEV1/FVC relationship obtained with the predicted values of four different ethnic groups in subjects with different age, sex and ventilatory function (see text for explanation). The line represents the regression line for these data.

Figure 9-3 shows FVC isopleths for FVC values from 1.5 L to 5.5 L at intervals of FVC of 0.5 L. Each line was drawn estimating the FEF$_{25-75\%}$ values for a range of FEV1 from FEV1 = 70% of FVC up to FEV1 = FVC. Exceptions to this upper limit are isopleths for FVC values of 3.5 L or bigger, where the maximal value of FEV1 used was the one yielding an estimated FEF$_{25-75\%}$ =5 L/s, that was arbitrarily set as the upper limit for the y axis.

SPIROMETRY

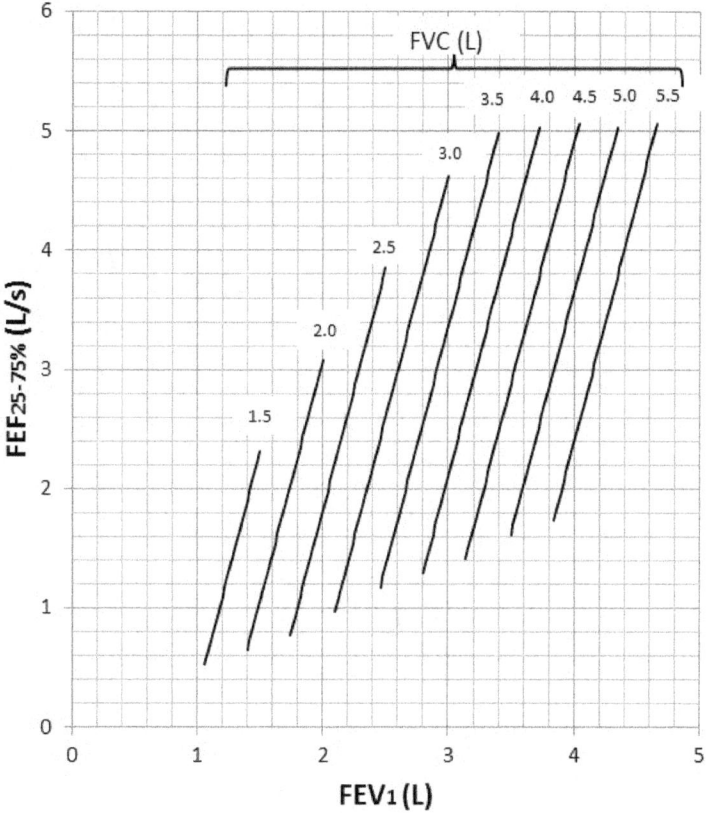

Figure 9-3. Group of FVC isopleths (constant FVC in each line) in the FEF25-75% vs. FEV1 relationship. On top of each line is written the value of FVC represented by the line.

Also, using a procedure similar to the one applied to the exponential equation in the previous chapter (see Table 8-1), it was possible to draw lines representing the same value of FEV_1/FVC (isoFEV$_1$/FVC lines or FEV$_1$/FVC isopleths). Figure 9-4 shows isoFEV$_1$/FVC lines for FEV$_1$/FVC values of 0.7, 0.8 and 0.9.

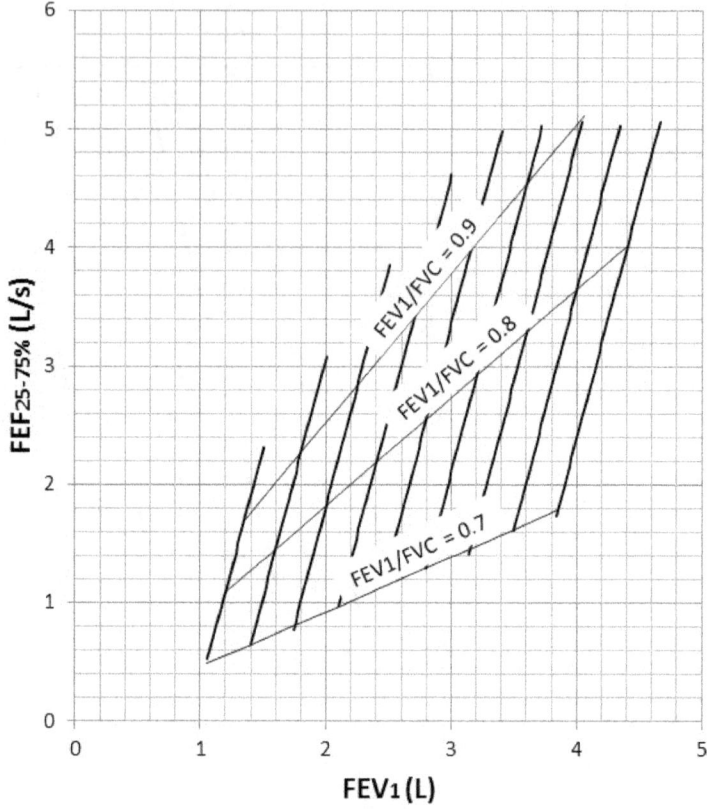

Figure 9-4. The FEF25-75%-FEV1 diagram showing a group of FVC isopleths and FEV1/FVC isopleths within the range of predicted values.

The graph shown in Figure 9-4 can be called the FEF25-75%-FEV1 diagram for predicted values. It represents approximately the interrelationships among the main spirometry parameters within predicted values of the four ethnic groups considered in the analysis. The graph may be helpful for showing longitudinal changes of the spirometry parameters simultaneously in one graph. For example, as was mentioned earlier in this chapter, the calculated 120 sets of predicted values can be considered predicted values for a longitudinal study of 8 subjects from age 8 to 80. Using the sets of spirometry parameters corresponding to a male Caucasian during that age span, it is possible to represent in the graph the calculated predicted values from age 8 to 80 and graphically observe the evolution of predicted lung function with age, as shown in Figure 9-5.

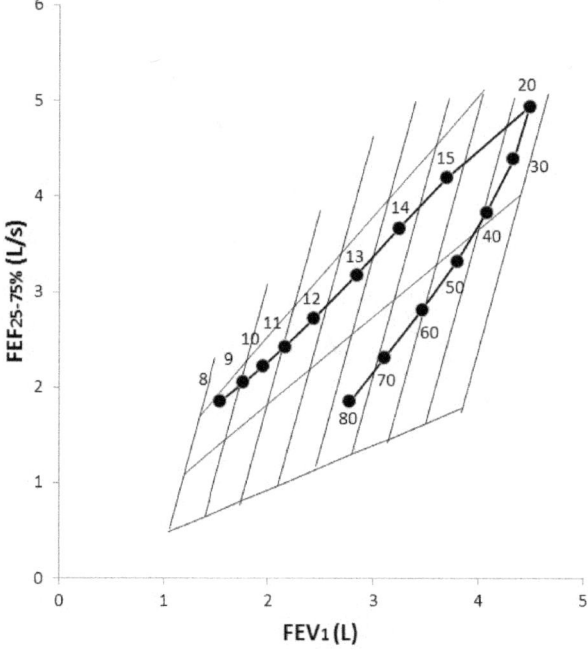

Figure 9-5. Graphical representation of the longitudinal changes in predicted spirometry parameters for a Caucasian male from 8 to 80 years old (see text for the values of height that were used in the calculations). The number at the side of each point represents the age of the subject at that point.

It is interesting to observe that, for a given value of forced vital capacity, the maximal expiratory flow is lower when lung function decreases with age than during the increase in lung function during the growing period.

In the same way, it is possible to graphically observe and compare the evolution of predicted lung function with age for male subjects of the four ethnic groups considered in the analysis, as shown in Figure 9-6.

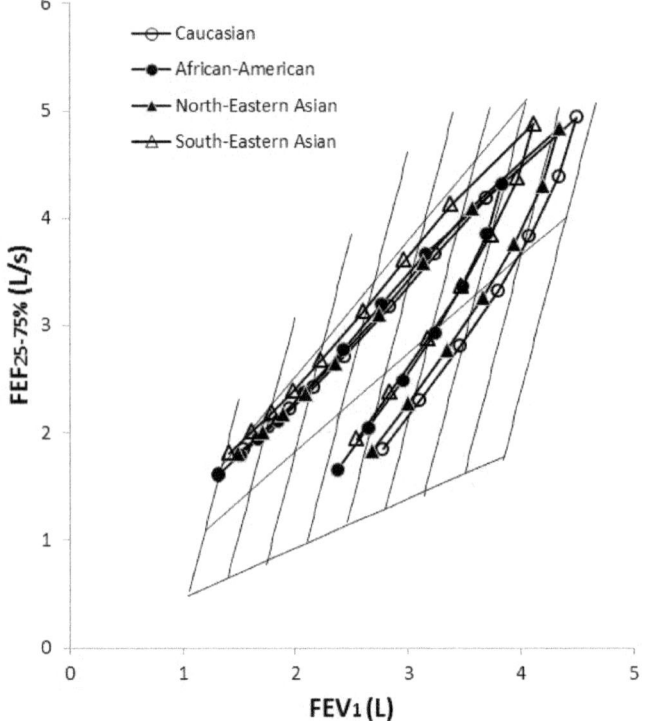

Figure 9-6. Graphical representation of the longitudinal changes in predicted spirometry parameters for males of the four ethnic groups from 8 to 80 years old (see text for the values of height that were used in the calculations).

Chapter 10

INTERRELATIONSHIP OF SPIROMETRY PARAMETERS: PRACTICAL APPLICATIONS

"The failure to distinguish between FEV_1 as a sign of obstruction and FEV_1 as a marker of a low FVC has caused great confusion, much of which has arisen from a failure to measure or report the FVC."

The above sentence was taken from an editorial of Peter Burney[50] commenting about a study on changes in FEV_1 over time in patients with chronic obstructive pulmonary disease (COPD).[51] Those words represent a practical application of the interrelationship of spirometry parameters, reminding us that the interpretation of changes in FEV_1 should be analyzed in the context of simultaneous changes in FVC.

The aging process of the lungs is an example of a situation in which a decrease in FEV_1 is partly due to a decrease in maximal expiratory flow rate, but it is also due to a decrease in FVC. For example, in a Caucasian male subject with a height of 175 cm, the predicted values from age 30 to 80 years are those shown in Table 10.1.

Using equation 1 from Chapter 9, it is possible to estimate

which would be the values of FEV1 if FVC stayed constant while the maximal expiratory flow decreases as a result of the aging process. These estimations are shown in Table 10-2.

Table 10-1. Predicted values for a Caucasian male with 175 cm of height.

Age (yr.)	FVC (L)	FEV1 (L)	FEF25-75% (L/s)
30	5.24	4.33	4.39
40	5.05	4.08	3.83
50	4.80	3.80	3.32
60	4.47	3.46	2.81
70	4.09	3.10	2.30
80	3.75	2.78	1.85

Table 10-2. Estimated values FEV1 for the Caucasian male in Table 10-1 if FVC stayed constant as the maximal expiratory flow decreases with age.

Age (yr.)	FVC (L)	FEV1 (L)	FEF25-75% (L/s)
30	5.24	4,33	4.39
40	5.24	4,20	3.83
50	5.24	4,07	3.32
60	5.24	3,95	2.81
70	5.24	3,82	2.30
80	5.24	3,71	1.85

SPIROMETRY

Data of FEV1 and FEF25-75% from Tables 10-1 and 10-2 are graphically represented in Figure 10-1 (straight lines in the figure representing constant values of FVC are only approximations; see Figure 9-3). If FVC stayed constant with age, the decrease in FEV1 would follow the trajectory of an FVC isopleth (a line representing constant FVC, from A to B) (Table 10-2). However, from age 30 to 80 years, predicted FEV1 decreases from 4.33 L to 2.78 L, but FVC also decreases from 5.24 L to 3.75 L, that is, from A to C (Table 10-1).

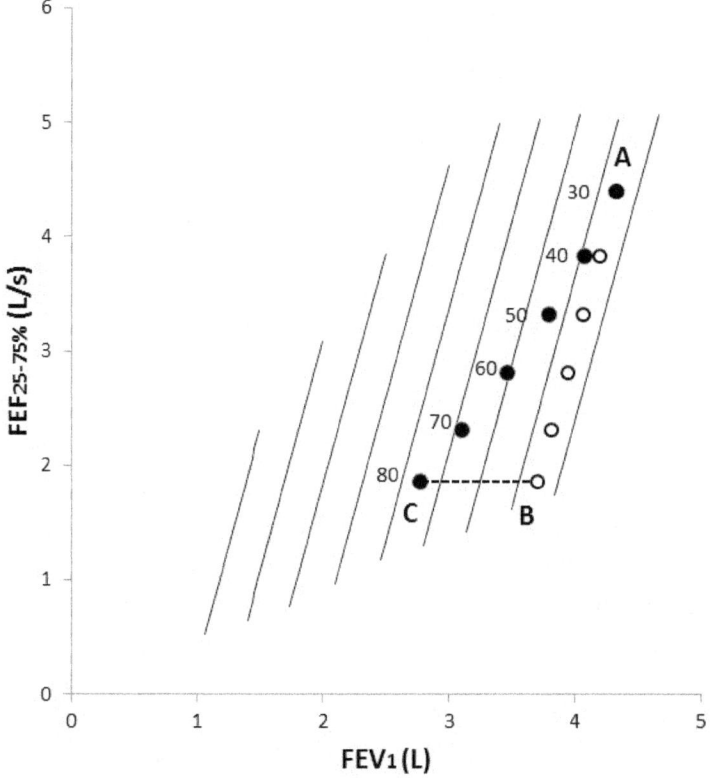

Figure 10-1. Graphic representation of data in Tables 10-1 (dots) and 10-2 (open circles). The dotted line represents the decrease in FEV1 with age due to a decrease in FVC. Numbers represent the age of the subject at each point.

If FVC stayed constant with age, FEV_1 would decrease only to 3.71 L (Table 10-2). That is, of the 1.55 L total decrease in predicted FEV_1 (4.33 - 2.78 = 1.55) from age 30 to 80, approximately 0.62 L (4.33 - 3.71 = 0.62), is due to a decrease in maximal expiratory flow rate, and the rest, approximately 0.93 L (3.71 -2.78 = 0.93), is due to a decrease in FVC.

In the same way that any change in FVC must be considered to evaluate a change in FEV_1, changes in $FEF_{25-75\%}$ should not be judged without taking into account possible changes in FVC. Using similar words to those shown at the beginning of this chapter, it can be said that the failure to distinguish between changes in $FEF_{25-75\%}$ as a sign of obstruction and changes in $FEF_{25-75\%}$ as a consequence of variations in FVC has caused great confusion, much of which has arisen from a failure to measure or report the FVC.

Spirometry changes that may occur in lung transplant recipients represent a good example to illustrate the importance of taking into consideration variations in FVC when analyzing changes in $FEF_{25-75\%}$.

The follow-up of ventilatory function changes in lung transplant recipients is essential for detecting the occurrence of the Bronchiolitis Obliterans Syndrome (BOS). The current grading system for BOS uses both FEV_1 and $FEF_{25-75\%}$ to define a zero-potential-BOS stage (BOS 0-p) which is characterized by a 10% to 19% decrease in FEV_1 and/or by a $\geq$ 25% decrease in $FEF_{25-75\%}$ from baseline.[52,53] The addition of $FEF_{25-75\%}$ to the original staging system[52] was due to studies showing that $FEF_{25-75\%}$ was more sensitive than FEV_1 for early detection of airway obstruction in BOS.[54-56] However, more recent studies seem to contradict the higher sensitivity of $FEF_{25-75\%}$. The FEV_1 criterion was found to be a better predictor of BOS stage 1 than the $FEF_{25-75\%}$ criterion after bilateral and single-lung transplantation.[57,58]

There is no contradiction between studies claiming a higher sensitivity either of FEV_1 or $FEF_{25-75\%}$ to detect BOS, and both criteria can be reconciled. In these studies, any decrease in FEV_1 or $FEF_{25-75\%}$ was considered a sign of airway obstruction. However, the variable dependence of $FEF_{25-75\%}$ on FVC, which is different from the dependence of FEV_1, was not taken into account. A change in FVC (increase or decrease) almost invariably results in a likewise change in FEV_1, but this is not the case for $FEF_{25-75\%}$. We can find situations in which both FEV_1 and $FEF_{25-75\%}$ change in the same direction of FVC. For example, let us look at the variation in ventilatory function with height comparing normal subjects with different height. The predicted spirometry parameters for a 30 years old Caucasian male subject with a height of 155 cm are: FVC= 3.91 L, FEV_1 = 3.31 L and $FEF_{25-75\%}$ = 3.62 L/s. For a subject with the same characteristics but a height of 170 cm, the predicted values are: FVC = 4.89 L, FEV_1 = 4.06 L and $FEF_{25-75\%}$ = 4.23 L/s. In this situation, a higher FVC is associated with higher values of both FEV_1 and $FEF_{25-75\%}$.

By contrast, we can also find situations in which an increase in FVC is followed also by an increase in FEV_1 with a decrease or no change in $FEF_{25-75\%}$. This is a common situation in post-bronchodilator spirometry tests. If FVC increases, post-bronchodilator $FEF_{25-75\%}$ is not comparable with the value measured before the bronchodilator (see Chapter 7).[36] An improved post-bronchodilator ventilatory function evidenced by increased FVC and FEV_1 is often associated with a decreased $FEF_{25-75\%}$ that is not a sign of worsening of the airway obstruction. The opposite to this situation can be observed in asthmatic patients with airway obstruction producing gas trapping and increased residual volume, simulating a restrictive defect.[59] These cases may present reduced FVC and FEV_1 but FEV_1/FVC within normal predicted values.

All changes in FVC, FEV_1 and $FEF_{25-75\%}$ described above can be visually analyzed with a $FEF_{25-75\%}$-FEV_1 diagram (Figure 10-2).

Taking as baseline values of ventilatory function those represented by a dot in Figure 10-2, horizontal dashed arrows show that FEV1 can increase or decrease in a subsequent test following likewise changes in FVC, and this without a change in FEF25-75%. This means that if both FVC and FEV1 decrease, FEF25-75% may be insensitive to the change in ventilatory function. Starting again from the baseline test in Figure 10-2, vertical dashed arrows show that FEF25-75% can change following opposite changes in FVC and no change is observed in FEV1. In other words, if FVC decreases and there is no change in FEV1 then FEF25-75% increases. By contrast, going in the opposite direction we observe that FEF25-75% may decrease only because FVC has increased, even in the absence of change in FEV1. Changes in the FEV1/FVC ratio have also occurred but they are not represented in the figure.

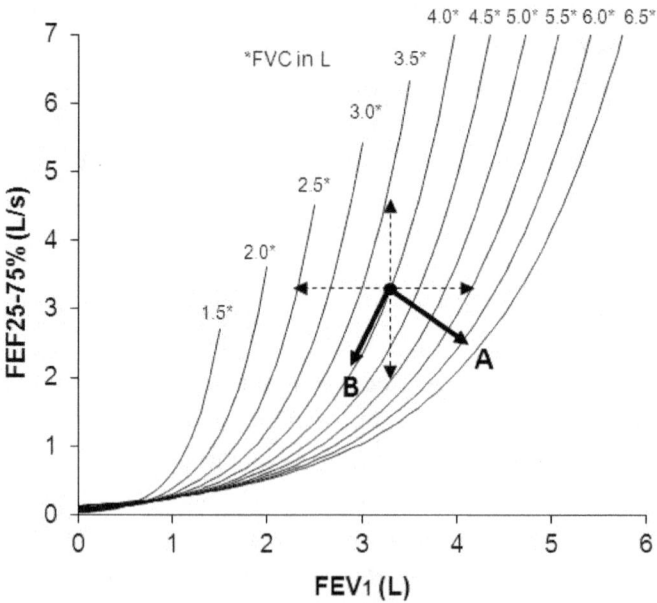

Figure 10-2. Graphic showing the interrelationship of spirometry parameters. See text for arrows' description.

SPIROMETRY

The thick arrow labeled with "A" in Figure 10-2 shows another situation in which $FEF_{25-75\%}$ decreases without any evidence of deterioration of the ventilatory function. In this case, both FVC and FEV_1 have increased. A patient with supra-normal $FEF_{25-75\%}$ soon after bilateral lung transplantation reported by Hachem and colleagues is an example of this situation.[57] The one month post-transplant spirometry parameters of the patient were: FVC = 2.61 L, FEV_1 = 2.60 L and $FEF_{25-75\%}$ = 9.94 L/s; the one year post-transplant parameters were: FVC = 3.90 L (increase of 49%), FEV_1 = 3.63 (increase of 40%) and $FEF_{25-75\%}$ = 5.96 L/s (decrease of 40%). In this case, the ventilatory function of the patient improved although there was a marked decrease in $FEF_{25-75\%}$. The definition of a zero-potential-BOS stage (BOS 0-p) characterized by a $\geq 25\%$ decrease in $FEF_{25-75\%}$ from baseline does not apply to this patient due to the great increase in FVC and FEV_1.

The thick arrow labeled with "B" in Figure 10-2 illustrates the situation in which both $FEF_{25-75\%}$ and FEV_1 decrease without any important change in FVC. A change in $FEF_{25-75\%}$ is expected to be of greater magnitude than a change in FEV_1 due to the exponential relationship between these parameters at constant FVC. In this situation, a change in $FEF_{25-75\%}$ is more sensitive than FEV_1 for early detection of airway obstruction, and the $FEF_{25-75\%}$ criterion for a potential-BOS stage outperforms the FEV_1 criterion in lung transplant recipients. Keller and colleagues[60] reported a patient that approximately followed this path of ventilatory changes just before confirming the presence of bronchiolitis obliterans (BO). The patient developed BOS following a heart-lung transplant for pulmonary hypertension, and the clinical diagnosis of BO was done at 21 months due to the persistent decline in $FEF_{25-75\%}$.[60] Figure 10-3 is the graphic display of patient's changes in a $FEF_{25-75\%}$ vs. FEV_1 diagram up to the moment when BO was histologically confirmed, 25 months after transplant.

In conclusion, the interpretation of a decrease in FEV_1 or in $FEF_{25-75\%}$ as sign of airway obstruction should not be made without analyzing simultaneous changes in FVC and FEV1/FVC. There are situations in which FEV1 is more sensitive than FEF25-75% to detect changes in the ventilatory function, mostly when FVC has also changed. When changes in ventilatory function do not importantly affect FVC, the FEF25-75% has greater sensitivity than FEV1 to detect the change.

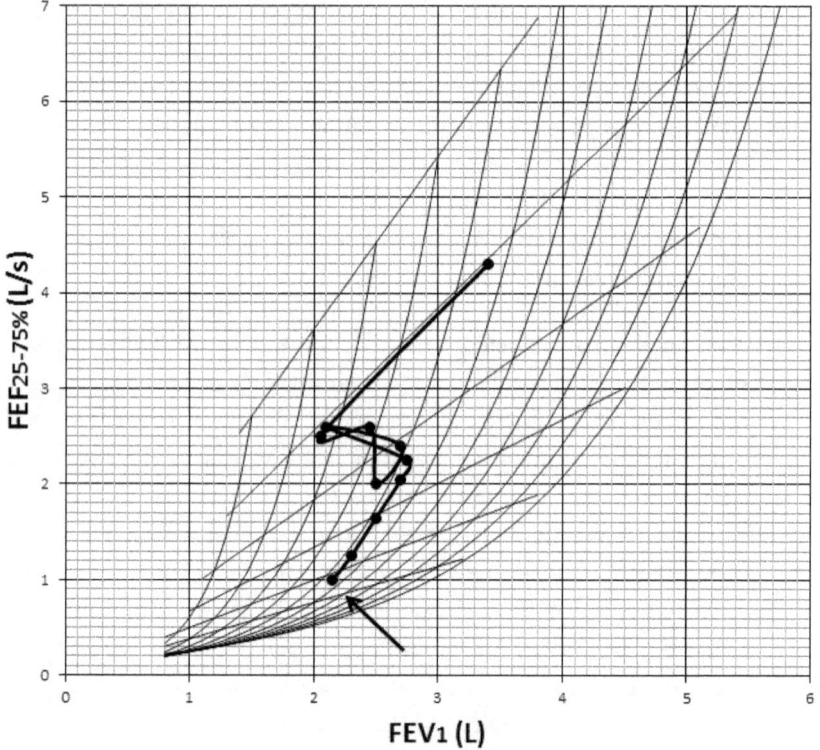

Figure 10-3. Changes in FEV1 and FEF25-75% reported by Keller and colleagues[60] in a heart-lung transplant recipient. The diagnosis of bronchiolitis obliterans was done due to the persistent decline in FEF25-75% (pointed by the arrow).

Chapter 11

STEP BY STEP ANALYSIS OF NUMERIC RESULTS

This chapter is dedicated to make an analysis, step by step, of the numeric results of a spirometry test. As explained in Chapter 5, the interpretation of spirometry tests includes the evaluation on the quality of the test, observation of the spirogram, and analysis of the numeric results. Assuming that the test is of good quality and no particular pattern of upper airway obstruction is observed in the flow-volume curve, the focus of this chapter is on the numeric results.

Analysis of the results of a spirometry test is made by comparing measured values with the appropriate predicted values and lower limits of normal (LLN) chosen according to the anthropometric characteristics of the subject. We may follow an interpretative strategy with a sequence of analysis or algorithm that leads to the final interpretation. Figure 11-1 shows the algorithm of an interpretative strategy. The interpretation strategy shown in Figure 11-1 is not the only one that can be followed. As mentioned before in Chapter 6, the interpretation is made after analyzing all parameters as a group to identify a particular spirometry pattern.

The analysis in this chapter is made taking into consideration the different situations that one may find during the interpretation. To follow the step by step interpretation described below, the reader may have in his/her hands the results of real spirometry tests as well as the predicted values and LLN of each parameter in order to practice the interpretation strategy while reading the chapter.

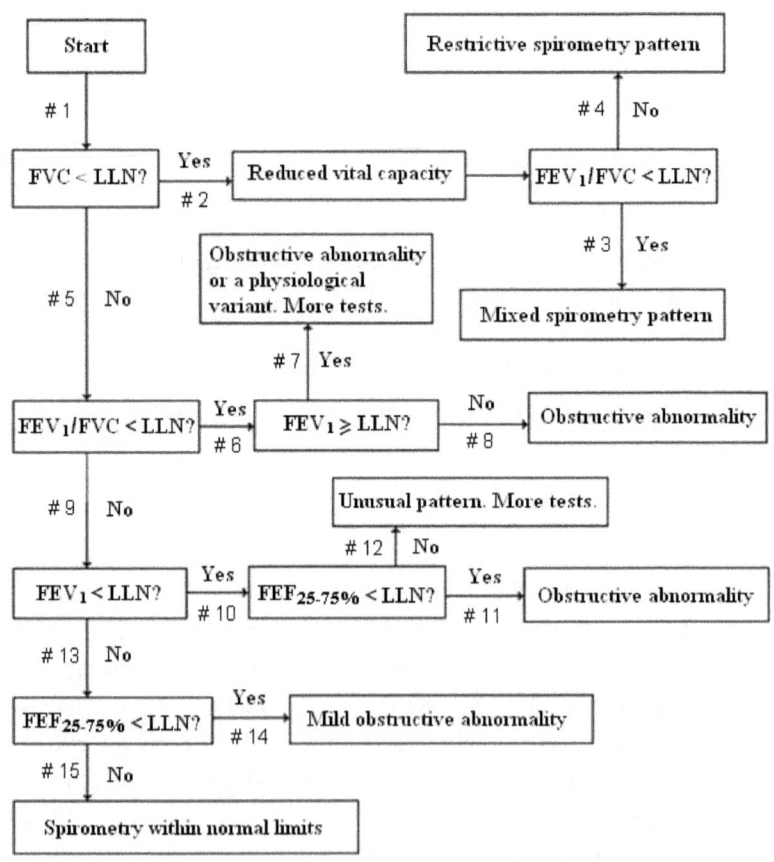

Figure 11-1. Algorithm of the interpretative strategy.

Step 1

Let us start by looking at FVC.

Is the measured FVC lower than the LLN?

No: go to Step 5

Yes: continue to Step 2

Step 2

As the FVC is lower than the LLN, the analysis of the parameters is leading us toward a restrictive spirometry pattern and the possible presence of a restrictive disorder. At this point, if the slow vital capacity (VC) has been also measured, it is better to take the highest measured value of vital capacity, FVC or VC (most probably it is the VC), and continue the analysis with the chosen value. If the measure of VC is available and it is at or above the LLN, then go to Step 5 and no longer take into consideration the restrictive pattern. If not, then continue within this Step 2.

As the vital capacity (FVC or VC) is reduced, a reduction in the absolute values of FEV_1 or $FEF_{25-75\%}$ could be simply the result of a smaller lung volume and, therefore, these two parameters are not taken into account in this situation. Next question:

Is the measured FEV_1/FVC (or FEV_1/VC) lower than the LLN?

No: go to Step 4

Yes: continue to Step 3

Step 3

Arriving to this point means that we are in front of a mixed spirometry pattern (see Table 6-4), with a restrictive component due to the reduced vital capacity and an obstructive component evidenced by the low FEV_1/FVC (or FEV_1/VC) ratio. It should be remembered that when there is a mixed spirometry pattern, in many cases the decrease in FVC is not due to a true restrictive abnormality or defect but to gas trapping as a consequence of airway obstruction. The spirometry test should be repeated after the administration of a bronchodilator for evaluating the reversibility of the ventilatory impairment.

Go to 'Final remark' at the end of the chapter.

Step 4

At this step, we are in front of a restrictive spirometry pattern (see Table 6-3), characterized by a reduced vital capacity without evidence of obstructive impairment because the FEV_1/FVC ratio is within normal limits. However, it should be remembered that the existence of a true restrictive defect cannot be assured only by spirometry. Clinical information may guide us in each particular case. If the spirometry test is the first respiratory test done on the subject, probably it is important to confirm or reject the presence of a true restrictive defect for diagnostic purposes. To do this, lung volumes should be measured, and particularly the total lung capacity. If the diagnosis of a restrictive defect (e.g. pulmonary fibrosis) has already been made in the patient, then the measurement of the vital capacity may give an idea of the magnitude of the ventilatory impairment. If the clinical information about the subject includes the diagnosis or suspicion of an obstructive disease then the spirometry test should be repeated after the administration of a bronchodilator. In such cases, a post-bronchodilator test may produce dramatic changes in the ventilatory function and change the spirometry pattern. For example, both FVC and FEV_1 may increase due to the opening of airways previously closed during the forced expiration. If a post-bronchodilator increase of FVC is proportionally greater than an increase of FEV_1, a post-bronchodilator obstructive spirometry pattern may be observed.

Go to 'Final remark' at the end of the chapter.

Step 5

Is the measured FEV$_1$/FVC lower than the LLN?

No: go to Step 9

Yes: continue to Step 6

Step 6

At this point, we are in front of a test with normal FVC and reduced FEV$_1$/FVC. In the vast majority of cases, this combination leads us to the conclusion of the presence of an obstructive ventilatory impairment. However, we should keep in mind that there are exceptions to the combination of normal FVC and reduced FEV$_1$/FVC. As mentioned in Chapter 6, there are subjects (usually with FVC above predicted) without respiratory problems showing this combination in the spirometry test. In front of a normal FVC and reduced FEV$_1$/FVC, to avoid providing a false positive result of the test, we should ask the following question:

Is FEV$_1$ at or above the LLN?

No: go to Step 8

Yes: continue to Step 7

Step 7

The spirometry pattern of normal FVC, decreased FEV$_1$/FVC, and normal FEV$_1$ can be the result of a mild obstructive abnormality but also it could be a physiological variant (see Table 6-6). Therefore, in these cases, it is important to evaluate the clinical information and other tests of respiratory function should be performed too. Interpretation of this pattern ends here.

Step 8

At this step, we have the spirometry pattern of normal FVC, decreased FEV_1/FVC, and FEV_1 below the LLN (see Table 6-5). This is the characteristic pattern of an obstructive abnormality.

Go to 'Final remark' at the end of the chapter.

Step 9

Arriving to this step means that both FVC and FEV_1/FVC, two basic parameters in spirometry interpretation, are within normal limits. There is no evidence of a restrictive pattern (FVC is normal) and no evidence of an obstructive impairment (FEV_1/FVC is normal). We should now evaluate the third basic parameter in spirometry: the FEV_1.

Is the measured FEV_1 lower than the LLN?

No: got to step 13

Yes: continue to step 10

Step 10

There seems to be a paradox when we arrive to this step. The FVC is normal, the proportional relationship between FEV_1 and FVC (i.e. the FEV_1/FVC ratio) is also normal, but FEV_1 is below the lower limit. For interpreting this spirometry pattern, we should take into account the measured value of $FEF_{25-75\%}$.

Is the measured $FEF_{25-75\%}$ lower than the LLN?

No: got to step 12

Yes: continue to step 11

Step 11

At this step, we have a spirometry pattern of normal values of FVC and FEV$_1$/FVC along with decreased values of FEV$_1$ and FEF$_{25\text{-}75\%}$ (see Table 6-8). As both FEV$_1$ and FEF$_{25\text{-}75\%}$ have followed the same tendency toward a decrease, we can arrive to the conclusion that this is the spirometry pattern of an obstructive abnormality, although FEV$_1$/FVC is within normal limits. Most probably, FEV$_1$/FVC is very close to or at the LLN.

Go to 'Final remark' at the end of the chapter.

Step 12

Arriving to this step means we have a spirometry pattern with normal values of FVC, FEV$_1$/FVC and FEF$_{25\text{-}75\%}$, along with decreased values of FEV$_1$ (see Table 6-9). This is an unusual spirometry pattern which could be the result of a test that was not well performed. However, we said at the beginning of this chapter that we are assuming we are analyzing good quality tests, thus we will drop the possibility of a bad test. This spirometry pattern is probably due to the installation of a restrictive impairment. The FVC is normal in this case, but most probably its value is very close to the LLN. In this case, FEV$_1$ and FEF$_{25\text{-}75\%}$ have not followed the expected proportional change observed when FVC does not change (see Figure 8-2); FEV$_1$ is decreased but the FEF$_{25\text{-}75\%}$ is still within normal limits. This situation can be observed when there is a decrease of FVC (see Figure 8-8). To analyze this situation, we should keep in mind that there is a range of normality for all parameters and that the LLN are not strict boundaries between normality and abnormality. This could be the spirometry pattern of an early restrictive defect in which FVC is lower than the predicted value but not below the LLN. The subject's evolution should be followed, and clinical data and other tests may orient to a definitive diagnosis. Interpretation of this pattern ends here.

Step 13

The three basic parameters of spirometry, FVC, FEV_1 and the FEV_1/FVC ratio, are within normal limits. Can we conclude that the test is normal? Many persons interpreting spirometry would stop the interpretation at this point and consider that the test is normal. In the opinion of this author, the interpretative process may be stopped at this point and conclude that the test is normal if the aim of the spirometry test is to pick up major functional abnormalities or for screening purposes.

However, subtle obstructive abnormality may also be evidenced by spirometry. An early diagnosis of an obstructive impairment may be important for many patients. For example, the observation of a very mild obstructive abnormality in a smoker or in a subject working in an environment potentially harmful for the respiratory system could represent the early stage of a chronic obstructive lung disease and an early intervention such as convincing the patient to quit smoking or changing the subject's workplace may dramatically change the prognosis.

Looking for subtle abnormalities, we could now observe the measured value of $FEF_{25-75\%}$. It should be mentioned here that there are authors who discourage any use of this parameter but, in the opinion of this author, it is a valuable parameter when we are aware of its relationship with the other parameters. A limitation of this parameter was already mentioned in Chapter 3: low absolute values of $FEF_{25-75\%}$ could be simply the result of a smaller lung volume (as happens with FEV_1). Therefore, low absolute values of $FEF_{25-75\%}$ are not used as evidence of airway obstruction when FVC is decreased, but this is not the case in this Step 13. We have arrived to this point because the spirogram shows normal values of FVC, FEV_1 and FEV_1/FVC. Next question:

Is the measured $FEF_{25-75\%}$ lower than the LLN?

No: got to step 15

Yes: continue to step 14

Step 14

The spirometry pattern of normal values of FVC, FEV_1 and FEV_1/FVC along with a decreased $FEF_{25-75\%}$ is observed when there are early changes in the lungs associated with airflow obstruction. Therefore, this is an obstructive spirometry pattern (see Table 6-7).

Go to 'Final remark' at the end of the chapter.

Step 15

Arriving to this step means that all spirometry parameters are within normal limits. This is the pattern of normal spirometry test.

Final remark

In the above analysis of the numeric results of spirometry tests, no severity classification of the impairments has been made in case of abnormalities. To complete the interpretation, the severity of the ventilatory abnormality should be determined based on the absolute value of FEV_1, as shown in Chapter 6 (see Table 6-10).

José Almirall

Chapter 12

INTERPRETATION EXERCISES

Interpretation exercises in the following pages take into account only the numeric values of the different spirometry parameters. A complete interpretation should also include a comment on the test performance and any pertinent comment arising from the inspection of the spirogram.

EXERCISE 1

Data
Age: 25
Sex: m
Height: 175 cm
Race/Ethnic group: Caucasian
Spirometry (BTPS)

	Pred*	LL	Meas	% Pred
FVC (L)	5.33	4.31	4.70	(88)
FEV_1/FVC (%)	84	73	82	-
FEV_1 (L)	4.45	3.60	3.85	(87)
$FEF_{25-75\%}$ (L/s)	4.62	3.07	3.57	-

* Pred = Predicted values ; LL = Lower Limits ; Meas = Measured ; %Pred = Percent of predicted value.

Analysis

Parameter	Measured value is below the lower limit?	
	yes	no
FVC (L)		x
FEV_1/FVC (%)		x
FEV_1 (L)		x
$FEF_{25-75\%}$ (L/s)		x
Interpretation	Normal spirometry test	

Interpretation
Spirometry within normal limits: all parameters are above the lower limit of normal.

SPIROMETRY

EXERCISE 2

Data
Age: 40
Sex: m
Height: 180 cm
Race/Ethnic group: African-American
Spirometry (BTPS)

	Pred	LL.	Meas	% Pred
FVC (L)	4.57	3.56	5.40	118
FEV_1/FVC (%)	81	71	**70**	-
FEV_1 (L)	3.70	2.84	3.78	102
$FEF_{25-75\%}$ (L/s)	3.65	1.91	4.12	-

Analysis

Parameter	Measured value is below the lower limit?	
	yes	no
FVC (L)		x
FEV_1/FVC (%)	x	
FEV_1 (L)		x
$FEF_{25-75\%}$ (L/s)	N/E*	
Interpretation	Mild obstructive abnormality or a physiological variant. More tests.	

* N/E = Not evaluated because FEV_1/FVC is below the lower limit. See Chapter 6 for explanation.

Interpretation
The combination of FEV_1/FVC below the normal range along with normal FEV_1 is a pattern that can be seen in subjects with mild obstructive abnormality but also in healthy subjects and it may be a physiological variant. Other tests should be made.

EXERCISE 3

Data
Age : 55
Sex : f
Height : 160 cm
Race/Ethnic group: North East Asian
Spirometry (BTPS)

	Pred	LL.	Meas	% Pred
FVC (L)	3.12	2.52	2.90	(93)
FEV_1/FVC (%)	81	71	**64**	-
FEV_1 (L)	2.51	1.94	**1.85**	(74)
$FEF_{25-75\%}$ (L/s)	2.26	1.22	**1.18**	-

Analysis

Parameter	Measured value is below the lower limit?	
	yes	no
FVC (L)		x
FEV_1/FVC (%)	x	
FEV_1 (L)	x	
$FEF_{25-75\%}$ (L/s)	N/E*	
Interpretation	Obstructive abnormality	

* N/E = Not evaluated because FEV_1/FVC is below the lower limit. See Chapter 6 for explanation.

Interpretation
The FEV_1/FVC ratio below the normal range indicates an obstructive abnormality. The FEV_1 at 70% of the predicted value indicates that the impairment is mild (FEV_1% pred. $\geq$ 70 %).

EXERCISE 4

Data
Age : 40
Sex : m
Height : 170
Race/Ethnic group: Caucasian
Spirometry (BTPS)

	Pred	LL	Meas	% Pred
FVC (L)	4.71	3.75	4.63	(98)
FEV$_1$/FVC (%)	81	71	73	-
FEV$_1$ (L)	3.82	3.03	3.38	(88)
FEF$_{25\text{-}75\%}$ (L/s)	3.81	2.22	**2.09**	-

Analysis

Parameter	Measured value is below the lower limit?	
	yes	no
FVC (L)		x
FEV$_1$/FVC (%)		x
FEV$_1$ (L)		x
FEF$_{25\text{-}75\%}$ (L/s)	x	
Interpretation	Obstructive abnormality	

Interpretation
The maximal mid-expiratory flow (FEF$_{25\text{-}75\%}$) below the lower limit of normal indicates the presence of mild bronchial obstruction (FEV$_1$% pred. $\geq$ 70 %).

EXERCISE 5

Data
Age : 50
Sex : f
Height : 160 cm
Race/Ethnic group: African-American
Spirometry (BTPS)

	Pred	LL	Meas	% Pred
FVC (L)	2.85	2.18	2.28	(80)
FEV_1/FVC (%)	81	70	70	-
FEV_1 (L)	2.31	1.74	**1.60**	(69)
$FEF_{25-75\%}$ (L/s)	2.36	1.15	**0.95**	-

Analysis

Parameter	Measured value is below the lower limit?	
	yes	no
FVC (L)		x
FEV_1/FVC (%)		x
FEV_1 (L)	x	
$FEF_{25-75\%}$ (L/s)	x	
Interpretation	Obstructive abnormality	

Interpretation
The FEV_1/FVC ratio is within normal limits, but the FEV_1 and the $FEF_{25-75\%}$ are below the lower limit of normal. These data suggest the presence of a mild obstructive functional abnormality (FEV_1% pred. $\geq$ 70 %).

SPIROMETRY

EXERCISE 6
Data
Age : 30
Sex : m
Height : 170 cm
Race/Ethnic group: South East Asian
Spirometry (BTPS)

	Pred	LL	Meas	% Pred
FVC (L)	4.35	3.47	**3.22**	(74)
FEV_1/FVC (%)	86	76	89	-
FEV_1 (L)	3.72	2.95	**2.86**	(77)
$FEF_{25-75\%}$ (L/s)	4.19	2.75	**1.94**	-

Analysis

Parameter	Measured value is below the lower limit?	
	yes	no
FVC (L)	x	
FEV_1/FVC (%)		x
FEV_1 (L)	N/E*	
$FEF_{25-75\%}$ (L/s)	N/E*	
Interpretation	Restrictive spirometry pattern suggesting a restrictive abnormality	

* N/E = Not evaluated because FVC is below the lower limit. See Chapter 6 for explanation.

Interpretation
The vital capacity below the lower limit of normal is interpreted as a reduction in the volume excursion of the lungs, graded in this case as mild (FEV_1% pred. $\geq$ 70 %). A reduced vital capacity suggests the presence of a restrictive disease. Measurement of the total lung capacity is necessary to confirm or reject this suggestion.

EXERCISE 7

Data
Age : 30
Sex : f
Height : 165 cm
Race/Ethnic group: Caucasian
Spirometry (BTPS)

	Pred	LL	Meas	% Pred
FVC (L)	3.93	3.14	**2.48**	(63)
FEV_1/FVC (%)	85	73	**70**	-
FEV_1 (L)	3.32	2.66	**1.73**	(52)
$FEF_{25-75\%}$ (L/s)	3.66	2.36	**1.72**	-

Analysis

Parameter	Measured value is below the lower limit?	
	yes	no
FVC (L)	x	
FEV_1/FVC (%)	x	
FEV_1 (L)	N/E*	
$FEF_{25-75\%}$ (L/s)	N/E*	
Interpretation	Mixed spirometry pattern	

* N/E = Not evaluated because FVC is below the lower limit. See Chapter 6 for explanation.

Interpretation
The FEV_1/FVC ratio below the normal range indicates an obstructive abnormality. The forced vital capacity is also below the normal range. The FEV_1 at 52% of the predicted value indicates that the ventilatory defect is moderately severe (FEV_1 % pred. between 50 % and 59 %). The reduced vital capacity may be explained by an increase in residual volume as a result of the obstructive abnormality rather than by the presence of a restrictive disease. Lung volumes measurement is necessary to distinguish between these two possibilities. A post-bronchodilator test should be performed.

SPIROMETRY

EXERCISE 8
Data
Age : 20
Sex : m
Height : 180 cm
Race/Ethnic group: African-American
Spirometry (BTPS)

	Pred	LL	Pre-bronchodilator Meas	%Pred	Post-bronchodilator Meas	%Pred
FVC (L)	4.77	3.80	4.43	(93)	4.56	(96)
FEV_1/FVC (%)	86	75	**57**	-	**60**	-
FEV_1 (L)	4.08	3.22	**2.53**	(62)	**2.72**	(67)
$FEF_{25-75\%}$ (L/s)	4.49	2.69	**2.12**	-	**2.32**	-

Analysis

Parameter	Pre-bronchodilator Measured value is below the lower limit?		Post-bronchodilator Measured value is below the lower limit?	
	yes	no	yes	no
FVC (L)		x		x
FEV_1/FVC (%)	x		x	
FEV_1 (L)	x		x	
$FEF_{25-75\%}$ (L/s)	N/E*		N/E*	
Interpretation	Obstructive abnormality		Obstructive abnormality	

* N/E = Not evaluated because FEV_1/FVC is below the lower limit. See Chapter 6 for explanation.

Interpretation

Pre-bronchodilator spirometry: The FEV_1/FVC ratio below the normal range indicates an obstructive abnormality. The FEV_1 at 62% of the predicted value indicates that the defect is moderate (FEV_1 % pred. is between 60 % and 69 %).

Post-bronchodilator spirometry: Changes in FVC and FEV_1 (less than 200 ml and /or less than 12%) are not significant. Obstructive abnormality is still graded as moderate.

José Almirall

EXERCISE 9
Data
Age : 30
Sex : m
Height : 175 cm
Race/Ethnic group: Nord East Asian
Spirometry (BTPS)

	Pred.	LL	Pre-bronchodilator Meas	%Pred	Post-bronchodilator Meas	%Pred
FVC (L)	5.04	4.42	5.39	(107)	5.50	(109)
FEV$_1$/FVC (%)	83	75	**53**	-	**61**	-
FEV$_1$ (L)	4.18	3.62	**2.85**	(68)	**3.35**	(80)
FEF$_{25-75\%}$ (L/s)	4.30	2.87	**2.65**	-	**2.78**	-

Analysis

Parameter	Pre-bronchodilator Measured value is below the lower limit?		Post-bronchodilator Measured value is below the lower limit?	
	yes	no	yes	no
FVC (L)		x		x
FEV$_1$/FVC (%)	x		x	
FEV$_1$ (L)	x		x	
FEF$_{25-75\%}$ (L/s)	N/E*		N/E*	
Interpretation	Obstructive abnormality		Obstructive abnormality	

* N/E = Not evaluated because FEV$_1$/FVC is below the lower limit. See Chapter 7 for explanation.

Interpretation

Pre-bronchodilator spirometry: The FEV$_1$/FVC ratio below the normal range indicates an obstructive abnormality. The FEV$_1$ at 68% of the predicted value indicates that the defect is moderate.

Post-bronchodilator spirometry: The change in FEV$_1$ of 18% (500 ml) is significant. The FEV$_1$/VC ratio is still below the normal range and indicates an obstructive abnormality. Post-bronchodilator obstructive abnormality is graded as mild (FEV$_1$% pred. $\geq$ 70 %).

SPIROMETRY

EXERCISE 10
Data
Age : 20
Sex : f
Height : 160 cm
Race/Ethnic group: Caucasian
Spirometry (BTPS)

	Pred	LL	Pre-bronchodilator Meas	Pre-bronchodilator %Pred	Post-bronchodilator Meas	Post-bronchodilator %Pred
FVC (L)	3.66	2.93	**2.62**	(72)	3.31	(90)
FEV$_1$/FVC (%)	89	77	83	-	**72**	-
FEV$_1$ (L)	3.22	2.59	**2.18**	(68)	**2.38**	(74)
FEF$_{25-75\%}$ (L/s)	3.85	2.57	**2.17**	-	**2.23**	-

Analysis

Parameter	Pre-bronchodilator Measured value is below the lower limit?		Post-bronchodilator Measured value is below the lower limit?	
	yes	no	yes	no
FVC (L)	x			x
FEV$_1$/FVC (%)		x	x	
FEV$_1$ (L)	N/E*		x	
FEF$_{25-75\%}$ (L/s)	N/E*		N/E**	
Interpretation	Restrictive pattern suggesting a restrictive abnormality		Obstructive abnormality	

* N/E = Not evaluated because FVC is below the lower limit. See Chapter 7 for explanation.
** N/E = Not evaluated because FEV$_1$/FVC is below the lower limit. See Chapter 7 for explanation.

Interpretation
Pre-bronchodilator spirometry: The vital capacity at below the normal range is interpreted as a restriction in the volume excursion of the lungs. A reduced vital capacity suggests the presence of a restrictive disease. The FEV$_1$/FVC ratio is in the normal range but below the predicted value. A mixed obstructive-reduced vital capacity pattern might be suspected when a reduced FVC is associated with a FEV$_1$/FVC value in the normal range below the predicted value,

rather than being at or above the predicted value, as often seen in true restrictive disorders. Clinical data may confirm this suspicion.

Post-bronchodilator spirometry: The change in FVC of 26% and of 690 ml is significant, except if it is due to a longer exhalation time. An obstructive pattern is now observed (FEV_1/FVC below the normal range). The obstructive abnormality is graded as mild (FEV_1% pred. $\geq$ 70 %). The value of vital capacity after the bronchodilator is within normal limits. This discards a restrictive abnormality. Hence, the pre-bronchodilator measurement of FVC below the lower limit of normal should have been the result of an increase in residual volume at the expense of the vital capacity.

REFERENCES

1. Hutchinson J. On the capacity of the lungs and on the respiratory function with view of establishing a precise and easy method of detecting diseases by the spirometer. Trans Med Chir Soc London. 1846;29:137-252.
2. Miller MR, Hankinson J, Brusasco V, et al. Standardisation of spirometry. Eur Respir J. 2005;26:319-338.
3. Macklem PT, Mead J. Resistance of central and peripheral airways measured by a retrograde catheter. J Appl Physiol. 1967;22:395-401.
4. Marin JM, Carrizo SJ, Gascon M, Sanchez A, Gallego B, Celli BR. Inspiratory capacity, dynamic hyperinflation, breathlessness, and exercise performance during the 6-minute-walk test in chronic obstructive pulmonary disease. Am J Respir Crit Care Med. 2001;163:1395-1399.
5. Celli B, ZuWallack R, Wang S, Kesten S. Improvement in resting inspiratory capacity and hyperinflation with tiotropium in COPD patients with increased static lung volumes. Chest. 2003;124:1743-1748.
6. Milic-Emili J, Grunstein MM. Drive and timing components of ventilation. Chest. 1976;70 (supplement):131S- 133S.
7. Bégin P, Grassino A. Inspiratory muscle dysfunction and chronic hypercapnia in chronic obstructive pulmonary disease. Am Rev Respir Dis. 1991;143(5 Pt 1):905-912.
8. Ewald FWJ, Tenholder MF, Waller RF. Analysis of the inspiratory flow-volume curve. Should it always precede the forced expiratory maneuver? Chest. 1994;106:814-818.
9. Molho M, Shulimzon T, Benzaray S, Katz I. Importance of inspiratory load in the assessment of severity of airways obstruction and its correlation with CO_2 retention in chronic obstructive pulmonary disease. Am Rev Respir Dis. 1993;147:45-49.
10. Demir T, Ikitimur HD, Koc N, Yildirim N. The role of FEV6 in the detection of airway obstruction. Respir Med. 2005;99(1):103-106.
11. Lamprecht B, Schirnhofer L, Tiefenbacher F, et al. Six-second spirometry for detection of airway obstruction: a

population-based study in Austria. Am J Respir Crit Care Med. 2007;176(5):460-464.
12. Hansen JE, Sun XG, Wasserman K. Should forced expiratory volume in six seconds replace forced vital capacity to detect airway obstruction? Eur Respir J. 2006;27(6):1244-1250.
13. Morris ZQ, Huda N, Burke RR. The diagnostic importance of a reduced FEV1/FEV6. COPD. 2012;9(1):22-28.
14. Hankinson JL, Crapo RO, Jensen RL. Spirometric reference values for the 6-s FVC maneuver. Chest. 2003;124:1805-1811.
15. Rao DR, Gaffin JM, Baxi SN, Sheehan WJ, Hoffman EB, Phipatanakul W. The utility of forced expiratory flow between 25% and 75% of vital capacity in predicting childhood asthma morbidity and severity. J Asthma. 2012;49(6):586-592.
16. Bégin P, Almirall J, Laprise C. Is forced expiratory flow between 25% and 75% of the forced vital capacity as a marker of airway obstruction redundant? [abstract]. Chest 2001;120 (suppl):292S-293S.
17. Gilbert R, Auchincloss JHJ. The interpretation of the spirogram. How accurate is it for 'obstruction'? Arch Intern Med. 1985;145:1635-1639.
18. Miller MR, Crapo R, Hankinson J, et al. General considerations for lung function testing. Eur Respir J. 2005;26:153-161.
19. American Thoracic Society. Standardization of spirometry: 1994 update. Am J Respir Crit Care Med. 1995;152:1107-1136.
20. Stoller JK, Basheda S, Laskowski D, et al. Trial of standard versus modified expiration to achieve end-of-test spirometry criteria. Am Rev Respir Dis. 1993;148:275-280.
21. Eisen EA, Dockery DW, Speizer FE, et al. The association between health status and the performance of excessively variable spirometry tests in a population-based study in 6 U.S. cities. Am Rev Respir Dis. 1987;136:1371-1376.
22. Eisen EA, Oliver LC, Christiani DC, et al. Effects of spirometry standards in two occupational cohorts. Am Rev Respir Dis. 1985;132:120-124.

23. Ng'an'ga LW, Ernst P, Jaakkola MS, et al. Spirometric lung function. Distribution and determinants of test failure in a young adult population. Am Rev Respir Dis. 1992;145:48-52.
24. Almirall J, Begin P. Exclusion spirometry: an initiative to increase lung function assessment in primary care. Can Respir J. 2004;11(3):195-196.
25. Teklu B, Pierson DJ, Fair K, Schoene RB. The match test revisited. Blowing out a candle as a screening test for airflow obstruction. J Fam Pract. 1990;31:557-558, 561-552.
26. Snider TI, Stevens JP, Wilner FM, Lewis BM. Simple bedside test of respiratory function. J Am Med Assoc. 1959;170:1631-1632.
27. Olsen CR. The match test. A measure of ventilatory function. Am Rev Respir Dis. 1962;86:37-40.
28. Carilli AD, Henderson JR. Estimation of ventilatory function by blowing out a match. Am Rev Respir Dis. 1964;89:680-686.
29. Mead J. Dysanapsis in normal lungs assessed by the relationship between maximal flow, static recoil, and vital capacity. Am Rev Respir Dis. 1980;121:339-342.
30. Heathcote KL, Cockcroft DW, Fladeland DA, Fenton ME. Normal expiratory flow rate and lung volumes in patients with combined emphysema and interstitial lung disease: a case series and literature review. Can Respir J. 2011;18(5):e73-76.
31. American Thoracic Society. Standardization of spirometry: 1987 update. Am Rev Respir Dis. 1987;136:1285- 1298.
32. Miller RD, Hyatt RE. Evaluation of obstructing lesions of the trachea and larynx by flow-volume loops. Am Rev Respir Dis. 1973;108:475- 481.
33. Takishima T, Grimby G, Graham W, Knudson R, Macklem PT, Mead J. Flow-volume curves during quiet breathing, maximum voluntary ventilation, and forced vital capacities in patients with obstructive lung disease. Scand J Respir Dis. 1967;48:384-393.
34. Meysman M, Noppen M, Vincken W. Effect of posture on the flow-volume loop in two patients with euthyroid goiter. Chest 1996;110:1615- 1618.

35. American Thoracic Society. Lung function testing: selection of reference values and interpretative strategies. Am Rev Respir Dis 1991;144:1202-1218.
36. Pellegrino R, Viegi G, Brusasco V, et al. Interpretative strategies for lung function tests. Eur Respir J. 2005;26:948-968.
37. Stanojevic S, Wade A, Stocks J, et al. Reference ranges for spirometry across all ages: a new approach. Am J Respir Crit Care Med. 2008;177(3):253-260.
38. Quanjer PH, Stanojevic S, Cole TJ, et al. Multi-ethnic reference values for spirometry for the 3-95-yr age range: the global lung function 2012 equations. Eur Respir J. 2012;40(6):1324-1343.
39. Aaron SD, Dales RE, Cardinal P. How accurate is spirometry at predicting restrictive pulmonary impairment? Chest 1999;115:869-873.
40. Shapiro W, Patterson JLJ. Effects of smoking and athletic conditioning on ventilatory mechanics, including observations on the reliability of the forced expirogram. Am Rev Respir Dis. 1962;85:191-199.
41. Barisione G, Crimi E, Bartolini S, et al. How to interpret reduced forced expiratory volume in 1 s (FEV1)/vital capacity ratio with normal FEV1. Eur Respir J. 2009;33(6):1396-1402.
42. Kotti GH, Bell DG, Matthews T, Lucero PF, Morris MJ. Correlation of airway hyper-responsiveness with obstructive spirometric indices and FEV(1) > 90% of predicted. Respir Care. 2012;57(4):565-571.
43. Almirall JJ, Paez I. Interpretation of spirometric tests of asthmatic patients with reduced forced vital capacity. J Invest Allergol Clin Immunol. 1994;4:258- 260.
44. Jung YJ, Ra SW, Lee SD, Park CS, Oh YM. Clinical features of subjects with an isolated FEV1 reduction. Int J Tuberc Lung Dis. 2012;16(2):262-267.
45. Brand PLP, Quanjer PH, Postma DS, et al. Interpretation of bronchodilator response in patients with obstructive airways disease. Thorax 1992;47:429-436.
46. Rodríguez-Carballeira M, Heredia JL, Rué M, Quintana S, Almagro P. The bronchodilator test in chronic obstructive

pulmonary disease: Interpretation methods. Respiratory Medicine. 2007;101:34-42.
47. Olsen CR, Hale FC. A method for interpreting acute response to bronchodilators from the spirogram. Am Rev Respir Dis. 1968;98:301 302.
48. Pauwels RA, Buist AS, Calverley PM, Jenkins CR, Hurd SS, GOLD Scientific Committee. Global strategy for the diagnosis, management, and prevention of chronic obstructive pulmonary disease. NHLBI/WHO Global Initiative for Chronic Obstructive Lung Disease (GOLD) Workshop summary. Am J Respir Crit Care Med. 2001;163:1256-1276.
49. Tager IB, Weiss ST, Muñoz A, Welty C, Speizer FE. Determinants of response to Eucapnic hyperventilation with cold air in a population-based study. Am Rev Respir Dis. 1986;134:502-508.
50. Burney P. Variable loss of lung function in COPD. N Engl J Med. 2011;365(13):1246-1247.
51. Vestbo J, Edwards LD, Scanlon PD, et al. Changes in forced expiratory volume in 1 second over time in COPD. N Engl J Med. 2011;365(13):1184-1192.
52. Estenne M, Maurer JR, Boehler A, et al. Bronchiolitis obliterans syndrome 2001: An update of the diagnostic criteria. J Heart Lung Transplant. 2002;21:297-310.
53. Kotloff RM, Thabut G. Lung transplantation. Am J Respir Crit Care Med. 2011;184(2):159-171.
54. Reynaud-Gaubert M, Thomas P, Badier M, Cau P, Giudicelli R, Fuentes P. Early detection of airway involvement in obliterative bronchiolitis after lung transplantation. Functional and bronchoalveolar lavage cell findings. Am J Respir Crit Care Med. 2000;161:1924-1929.
55. Patterson GM, Wilson S, Whang JL, et al. Physiologic definitions of obliterative bronchiolitis in heart-lung and double lung transplantation: a comparison of the forced expiratory flow between 25% and 75% of the forced vital capacity and forced expiratory volume in one second. J Heart Lung Transplant. 1996;15:175-181.
56. Estenne M, Van Muylem A, Knoop C, Antoine M. Detection of obliterative bronchiolitis after lung

transplantation by indexes of ventilation distribution. Am J Respir Crit Care Med. 2000;162:1047–1051.
57. Hachem RR, Chakinala MM, Yusen RD, et al. The predictive value of bronchiolitis obliterans syndrome stage 0-p. Am J Respir Crit Care Med. 2004;169:468-472.
58. Lama VN, Murray S, Mumford JA, et al. Prognostic value of bronchiolitis obliterans syndrome stage 0-p in single-lung transplant recipients. Am J Respir Crit Care Med. 2005;172:379-383.
59. Colp C, Williams MHJ. Total occlusion of airways producing a restrictive pattern of ventilatory impairment. Am Rev Respir Dis. 1973;108:118- 122.
60. Keller CA, Cagle PT, Brown RW, Noon G, Frost AE. Bronchiolitis obliterans in recipients of single, double, and heart-lung transplantation. Chest. 1995;107:973-980.

APPENDIX

BTPS CORRECTION

Boyle's law states that, at a constant temperature, the volume of any gas varies inversely as the pressure to which the gas is submitted. In isothermal conditions, changing from pressure P_1 and volume V_1 to pressure P_1 and volume V_2, we have that $P_1 V_1 = P_2 V_2$.

Charles' law states that the volume of a gas at constant pressure increases proportionately to the absolute temperature. If V_1 and V_2 are volumes of the same mass of gas at absolute temperatures T_1 and T_2 then $V_1/V_2 = T_1/T_2$. Boyle's law and Charles' law may be combined as follows:

$$\frac{P_1 V_1}{T_1} = \frac{P_2 V_2}{T_2} \qquad \text{equation 1}$$

Because the number of water molecules in a wet gas varies with temperature and total pressure, the following form of Boyle's and Charles' laws is required for wet gas:

$$\frac{(P_1 - P_1(H_2O)) V_1}{T_1} = \frac{(P_2 - P_2(H_2O)) V_2}{T_2} \qquad \text{equation 2}$$

where $P_1(H_2O)$ and $P_2(H_2O)$ are the water vapor tensions under conditions 1 and 2 respectively.

In studies of respiratory function, if the actual expired gas measurement is made in a calibrated container (volume sensing device) at room temperature or with an unheated flow sensing device then the gas is under variable room (ambient) conditions, where the total pressure is the actual barometric pressure and the temperature is the temperature of the gas in the sensing device. These conditions are abbreviated ATPS (Ambient Temperature Pressure Saturated).

In measuring lung volumes, it is important to determine the quantity of space occupied by the gas when it was in the body. The observed ATPS volumes must therefore be corrected back to conditions prevailing in the lungs. The conventional "body conditions" are body temperature (which is assumed 37 degrees Celsius unless body temperature is abnormal), the actual barometric pressure, and saturated with water vapor (water vapor tension is 47 mmHg at temperature of 37 degrees C. These conditions are commonly abbreviated BTPS (Body Temperature Pressure Saturated).

If the subscript 1 in equation 2 represents BTPS conditions and subscript 2 represents ATPS conditions then,

$$\frac{(P_B - 47) \, V \text{ at BTPS}}{273 + 37} = \frac{(P_B - P(H_2O)) \, V \text{ at ATPS}}{273 + t} \quad \text{equation 3}$$

where V is the volume of gas, P_B is the barometric pressure, t is the ambient pressure in degrees Celsius, and $P(H_2O)$ is the water vapor tension at temperature t.

Solving equation 3 for V at BTPS we have,

$$V \text{ at BTPS} = V \text{ at ATPS} \times \frac{(P_B - P(H_2O))}{(P_B - 47)} \times \frac{273 + 37}{273 + t} \quad \text{equation 4}$$

INDEX

References to terms in figures are followed by an 'f'.

acceptability criteria, 37, 38
acini, 11, 12
airflow limitation, 35, 75
airway obstruction, 31-5, 45, 52, 54, 56, 62, 64-6, 68-69, 72-3, 75, 77, 79-80, 104-5 107, 109, 112, 116
alveolar sacs, 11, 12
alveoli, 11-2, 14, 18, 79
Ambient Temperature Pressure Saturated (ATPS), 9, 138
American Thoracic Society (ATS), 37, 43, 56, 73, 75
anatomical dead space, 12
anemometers, 6
asthma, asthmatic, 33, 40, 46, 66, 69-70, 75-6, 79, 105
ATPS, see Ambient Temperature Pressure Saturated
ATS, see American Thoracic Society
biological variation, 43-4
Body Temperature Pressure Saturated (BTPS), 8-9, 16, 138
bronchodilator response, 75, 77, 79
bronchospasm, 39
BTPS, see Body Temperature Pressure Saturated
bulk flow, 13
chronic obstructive pulmonary disease, 17, 20, 32, 53, 66, 76, 79, 101
CO_2 elimination, 18
conducting airways, 11-2
COPD, see chronic obstructive pulmonary disease
differential pressure flow, 6-7
diffuse airway obstruction, 52, 54
diffusion, 13
dynamic compression of the airways, 25, 30, 66
effort-dependent, 24
effort-independent, 24
emphysema, 13, 27, 47
end-expiratory position, 13, 17
equal pressure points, 25
ERS, see European Respiratory Society
ERV, see expiratory reserve volume
European Respiratory Society, 37, 43, 56, 73, 75
expiratory flow limitation, 24, 27, 30, 66
expiratory reserve volume (ERV), 16f, 17

extrathoracic, 27, 55-6
FEF$_{25-75\%}$, 32-4, 34f, 57, 59, 61, 63-71, 77, 78f, 81-2, 84-5, 85f, 86f, 87f, 88-9, 89f, 90f, 93-6, 97f, 98f, 98, 102-8, 108f, 111, 114-7
FEF$_{25-75\%}$/FVC, 81-3, 83f, 86, 94, 95f,
FEF$_{25-75\%6}$, 34
FEF$_{25\%}$, 36
FEF$_{50\%}$, 36
FEF$_{75\%}$, 36
FEV$_1$, 31, 33-4, 38-41, 53, 56, 59, 61-76, 79, 81, 84, 85f, 85, 86f, 87f, 88-9, 89f, 90f, 91f, 93, 95-6, 97f, 98f, 98, 101-8, 111-7
FEV$_1$/FVC, 31, 33, 35, 56, 59, 61-72, 79, 81-2, 83f, 84, 85, 88-9, 90f, 91f, 94-5, 95f, 96f, 97, 98f, 105-6, 108, 111-7
FEV$_1$/VC, 70, 111-2, 128
FEV$_6$, 31-2, 34-5
Fleisch pneumotachograph, 7, 8f
flow-sensing devices, 5-6, 9
flow-volume curve, 4, 22-3, 23f, 27, 35, 36f, 53, 73, 109
forced expiration, 5, 15, 21-2 24, 26, 29, 31, 33, 35, 37, 46, 53f, 54f, 56, 112
forced expiratory maneuver, 22, 22f, 23, 23f, 24-6, 26f, 29, 31-2, 35, 37-8, 53
forced expiratory volume in time interval t, see FEVt
forced inspiratory maneuver, 25-6, 26f, 27
forced vital capacity, see FVC
FRC, 16f, 17, 19, 26
Functional residual capacity, see FRC
FVC, 22-3, 29-36, 38-9, 56-7, 59, 61-73, 75-7, 81-2, 84-5, 85f, 86f, 86, 87f, 88-9, 90f, 91f, 93-6, 97f, 98f, 101-8, 111-7
FVC$_6$, 32
gas trapping, 65-6, 70, 105, 112
IC, 16f, 17
inspiratory capacity, see IC
inspiratory time, 19
inspiratory reserve volume, (IRV), 16f, 16-7
inter-individual variability, 44
interpretation exercises, 119-130
interrelationship, 81, 85f, 86, 87f, 89, 90f, 91f, 93, 98, 101, 106f
intra-individual variability, 44, 67
intrathoracic, 27, 55-6, 77
isovolume FEF$_{25-75\%}$, 77, 78f
kymograph, 4, 4f
kyphoscoliosis, 46
Lilly type pneumotachometers, 8
limitations of spirometry, 14, 47
lower limits of normal, 33, 60-2, 71, 109

maneuver of forced expiration, 26
maneuver of forced inspiration, 25
maximal expiratory flow-volume curve, 22, 23f, 53
maximal inspiratory flow-volume, 26
maximal voluntary ventilation, 20
maximum mid-expiratory flow rate, 32
MEFV, see maximal expiratory flow-volume curve
MIFV, see maximal inspiratory low-volume
minute ventilation, 14, 18, 20
mixed spirometry pattern, 65, 111-2, 126
MMFR, see maximum mid-expiratory flow rate
MVV, see maximal voluntary ventilation
O2 uptake, 18
obstruction of the major airways, 52, 55, 55f, 56
obstructive spirometry patterns, 66-7, 69-70, 112, 117
PEF, peak expiratory flow, 35, 37, 36f
performance of the test of forced expiration, 37, 53f
peripheral airway resistance, 13
persistent airway obstruction, 79
pleural pressure, 13, 24-5, 53

pneumotachographs, 6-8, 8f, 9
pneumotachometers, 6, 8
predicted values, 60, 62, 76, 79, 93-4, 95f, 96f, 98f, 98-9, 101, 102, 105, 109-10
pulmonary fibrosis, 15, 47, 112
pulmonary ventilation, 11, 13, 18, 20, 39
reference values, see predicted values
regional ventilation, 14
reproducibility criteria, 38-9
residual volume, 16f, 17, 23, 23f, 26f, 26, 27f, 66, 70, 77, 105, 126, 130
respiratory mechanics, 15, 66
restriction of lung excursion, 46-7
restrictive abnormality, 31, 47, 65, 73, 112, 125, 129-30
restrictive defect, 46, 62-4, 70-1, 105, 112, 115
restrictive pattern, 63-4, 111, 114
RV, see residual volume
severity classification, 72-4, 117
slow vital capacity, 70, 111
spirogram, 4, 15, 16f, 18, 21f, 21-2, 25, 29-31, 33, 38-9, 51, 53f, 63, 65, 69, 81, 109, 116, 119
spirometer, 3-4, 4f, 5, 6, 8-9, 15, 17, 22, 39-40, 43, 51, 56
spirometry interpretation, 51,

56, 59, 61, 63, 69, 72, 114
spirometry patterns, 35, 61-2,
  64-7, 69-72, 81, 89-90,
  109, 111-5, 117
spirometry tests, 4-5, 13-5,
  29, 37, 39, 44, 52, 57, 62,
  66, 79, 86, 105, 109-10,
  117
static lung volumes, 15, 30
technical variability, 43
test of forced expiration, 5,
  15, 21, 37, 40, 53f, 56
T_I/T_{tot}, 19
tidal volume, 16f, 16-18, 20
TLC, 16f, 18, 23f, 23, 26f,
  27f, 30, 62-4, 66, 77

total duration of a breathing
  cycle, 18
total lung capacity, see TLC
upper airway obstruction, 73,
  109 (see also obstruction
  of the major airways)
vital capacity (VC), 3, 4, 15,
  16f, 17, 23, 30-1, 35, 45-6,
  52, 70, 78f, 111
ventilation-perfusion
  relationship, 14
volume-sensing devices, 5
volume-time curve, 22f, 26f,
  29, 30f, 32, 34f, 52
V_T/T_I, 19

www.ingramcontent.com/pod-product-compliance
Lightning Source LLC
Chambersburg PA
CBHW071434180526
45170CB00001B/347